THE ART OF SENIOR DATING

HOW TO ATTRACT A TRAVEL COMPANION, TRUSTED FRIEND OR ROMANTIC PARTNER

RAVINA M CHANDRA

Published by RMC Publishers

ISBN 978-1-7775420-0-9 (Paperback)
ISBN 978-1-7775420-1-6 (Hardcover)
ISBN 978-1-7775420-4-7 (E-book)

www.ravinachandra.com

For all individuals wanting to live Vibrantly.
May your lives be fulfilling, balanced, and sparkly.

ALSO BY RAVINA M CHANDRA

In the *Inspired Retirement Living* Series

101 Ways to Enjoy Retirement
101 More Ways to Enjoy Retirement
101 Ways to Enjoy Retirement Across America

Other books

Longevity and Eating Habits
My Vibrant Life

TABLE OF CONTENTS

A SPECIAL GIFT JUST FOR YOU!

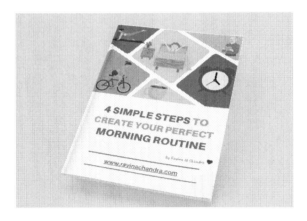

In '**4 Simple Steps to Create Your Perfect Morning Routine,**' you will discover:

- What a **morning routine** is and why it is essential you have one
- Why having a morning routine will bring you **more focus, productivity, and purpose to your life**
- The secret of creating a morning routine using these **four components** that will **align with your core values**
- How a morning routine can elevate your life so that you may live **vibrantly**, whether you are seeking a companion, exploring new interests, or improving your health

Go to www.ravinachandra.com/books to get it NOW

INTRODUCTION

How many evenings have loomed before you, seemingly endless as you try to fill them with tasks and mindless entertainment? By now, the allure of watching your favorite TV shows, reading, and doing puzzles has worn away. You've called a few friends, but they have plans with their partners, and you feel like an awkward third wheel.

As you watch a couple about your age walking by your house hand in hand, laughing and talking, you start to think, *'Maybe that could be me some day.'* You begin to picture yourself going out and meeting new people, but it just seems so overwhelming. Where do you start? What do you say? So much has changed since you went on your last date, and you don't even know the rules anymore.

I assure you that you can find someone to light up your life – on your terms.

There are people within a short walk or drive of you in the same situation who want just as eagerly to have companionship. But, like you, their social calendar also shows day after day of blank squares, and they just want to talk, laugh, and maybe share a little romance.

Your friends might be telling you to "Get out there and meet someone." If only it were that easy to find the right match!

First, you need to get your confidence up so you feel emotionally ready to meet new people and make sure they get to know the real you. If you've been on your own for a while or are used to sharing your life with one person, this can feel really daunting. Your married friends may not get it, but I do. Perhaps you've had a few relationships that haven't worked out the way you wanted. It's time to put all that baggage behind you. This is your fresh start, and you want to make the most of it.

To inspire you, think of the fun you'll have spinning on the dance floor with a trusted partner in your arms or competing playfully over a game of cribbage. Next, imagine picking up the phone to share that hilarious moment with your grandchild and laugh about it again as you tell the story to a person who really listens. Finally, picture yourself making plans that you can look forward to, forgetting about all those empty days you spent alone in your quiet home.

To help you ease into this next phase of your life, we're going to work through a twelve-week program that begins with two weeks of building your confidence, focusing on your positive traits, and assessing your physical and emotional state. This may include saying goodbye and letting go of past partners, or letting go of your grief over a lost love to free up your dynamic energy.

In weeks three and four, you'll build on that momentum by getting moving and clearing out the clutter from your home and your mind. We'll take small steps together that will really add up. By week five, you'll start defining what you truly want out of a relationship as you look ahead to your new life.

In the sixth week, you will begin practicing how to break the ice by getting out more and having different types of conversations before you start testing the waters. This will also make you feel more self-assured when the right moment arrives. In week seven, you will add a new weekly or biweekly activity to expand your network and meet new people.

In weeks eight and nine, we will look at whether or not online dating is for you, beginning with getting a flattering photo of you. Even if you never post your profile online, it's nice to summarize who you are in preparation for when you get introduced to a person you find attractive. At this point, you will discover where to find people who share your interests and values. This way, you will make fewer false starts and keep up that newfound confidence.

Honestly, you will make missteps along the way, but you will learn from them. To ease that process, I will share recommendations based on my own dating experiences and other sources, so that such missteps are less painful and maybe will even become a source of humor at some point. We are all learning, and this experience will be no different. You need to be patient as you sort through your feelings and the attributes of the people you meet in order to make the right match.

In week ten, we'll also make sure your search for a mate doesn't take up too much of your time, a common mistake of newbies to online dating, so you keep a balance in your life.

By week eleven, you will prepare for the possible awkward conversations about your aging bodies, your money, and your children's expectations. But, again, if you come to those discussions prepared and you are willing to stand up for yourself, they will unfold far more constructively, so you can focus on the more positive aspects of your time together. At this point, we assess what you've learned and how it will affect your next set of decisions.

By the time you've worked through the chapters of the book, as well as the twelve-week plan, my hope is that you will feel better about yourself, and this confidence will be reflected in the image you put out to the world. I'm actually going to ask you to document your 'before' and 'after' photos so you can see the difference. That's how much I believe in your ability to transform yourself and your life. In week twelve, we will celebrate how far you've come and how you feel about yourself now.

Don't worry. All these steps are outlined in a handy grid at the back of the book, and I'll be breaking them down one by one as we go through each chapter.

* * *

On a personal note, I am a successful career woman who was single throughout much of my life. I had almost given up on finding "the one" when I decided to do something about it a few years back. Out of pure necessity, I created a comprehensive, structured plan to get ready to find love, and I will take you on this same journey to prepare yourself for finding that companion or love interest.

Now, I am very happily married and am glad I waited for the man who truly makes me thrive in life. And I wish the same for you, whether you are seeking male or female companionship.

Additionally, I've spent more than twenty years working with older adults in the areas of health, nutrition, personal growth, and overall wellness, and I've noticed how loneliness, more often than not, plays such a significant role in each of these aspects. I've always really enjoyed encouraging others to be their best and have striven to help those ready to live a more vibrant life.

Most of all, I want you to enjoy the time you spend with the new people you meet along the way. So now, let's get started by introducing yourself to the new, vibrant you within.

WHY DATING IS POSSIBLE IN YOUR 60S, 70S (AND EVEN YOUR 80S)

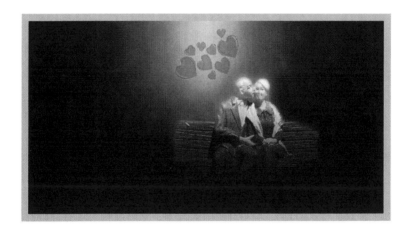

*W*hen you think of dating, you may flashback to the early days of your teens and twenties when people met at parties or while attending the same school or college. At that phase of your life, you could count on school, work, or friends to introduce you to new faces. You were expected to meet someone, settle down and focus on your career and family. However, these days, you are probably past all that, so there are fewer restrictions on what you can do with your time and energy. While this opens up some opportunities, it may also feel limiting, as you likely turn to the same circle of friends and your mutual connections. So, where do you start at this age to find someone who is compatible and wants the same things you do?

Rather than sit back and let the next several years just drift away, let's take a good look at what has changed and how that opens up so many possibilities for you.

The proportion of adults who are currently married is lower than it has ever been, as men and women seek out different types of companionship.[1] Over the past twenty-five years alone, the percentage of married men aged fifty years and older has dropped from 78 in 1990 to 67.3 in 2015. However, the rate for older women has barely changed from 52.6 percent to 52.7 percent over the same period. Fewer men are spending their later lives alone by being widowed (falling from 7.5 percent in 1990 to 5.7 percent in 2015), while levels of widowhood for women fell from 31.6 percent to 18.9 percent across the same period.

Divorce rates and the stigma attached to this type of separation have also changed dramatically. Between 1990 to 2015, the percentage of divorced men rose from 8.1 to 14.3, while the rates for women went from 10.1 to 18.1 percent in the United States.[2] Thirty years ago, divorce started becoming more acceptable as people left their unions, citing dissatisfaction as the main reason why they chose to move on with their lives in a new direction. In other words, more people began to acknowledge that leaving a relationship because you're unhappy doesn't make you a bad person. Instead, they simply wanted to seek out a new way of life, possibly with another shot at finding happiness and fulfillment. As a result, their quality of life actually improved after a divorce.

Similarly, the numbers of older adults who have never married have risen over the same period – 5 percent of men in 1990 versus 9.1 percent in 2015, and 4.9 percent of women versus 7.7 percent in 2015. Of course, some of those people are still single, but it doesn't mean they are not looking for love, just like I was. The same trend arises for couples who have lived in common-law unions. This type of arrangement more than doubled from 1.5 percent to 3.6 percent for men, and from less than 1 percent to 2.6 percent for women. These patterns tell us that traditional, lifelong marriage is no longer the norm for older adults.

SO, WHO IS OUT THERE?

The demographics for both the men and women available for dating and companionship have improved. Quite simply, life expectancy has increased, and now there is less of a gap between women and men. That means there are more men available for women to date. (Sorry guys, this may make it more competitive for you!)

As of 2017, in the United States, men lived on average to age 76.1 years, while women lived to 81.1 years. Some doctors believe this is due to women focusing more on their health in later life while men reward their longevity by enjoying rich foods and other treats they couldn't afford earlier in life. Thanks to advances in health care, the U.S. Census Bureau estimates that the average women's life expectancy will be 87.3 years by 2060, with men's at 83.9 years. Meanwhile, in Sweden, between 1997 and 2014, age-standardized all-cause mortality decreased by 26 percent in men and 16 percent in women, and life expectancy increased from 73.1 years to 76.1 years in men (rising by 3.0 years), and from 78.3 to 80.3 years in women (rising by 2 years).[3]

While people are generally living longer, they are also more active and doing things our parents would never think to try. Essentially, an eighty-year-old today is the new sixty-year-old. With better access to food and health care, we are more aware of how to live well, and it's paying off with vitality and a curiosity to explore and take on new ventures. You are more likely to have the income and outlook to explore the world, volunteer, or even still work if you love what you do. More seniors are doing activities once seen as only for young people, from skydiving to returning to university to keep their brains active.

Wouldn't that be even better if you didn't do it alone?

WHY AM I STILL SINGLE?

When you envisioned this part of your life, you may have imagined that you would be paired up before now. At this point, you can only foresee a future where you are stuck alone until the end of your days. However, your past doesn't need to dictate your future. There are many reasons why people are still unattached late in life, aside from long-standing relationships having ended. Let's look at why you are on your own and see if you can overcome some previous choices and habits. You may find that one or more of these sound familiar:

- **You waited for someone.** Maybe that other person was married, or you never recovered from a lover who chose to carry on without you. If you expect them to come back now, you're just losing valuable years that you could spend in a happy relationship with someone who appreciates you. After this long, it's time to release them from your life and stop comparing everyone else to them. Give yourself permission to start afresh without this person haunting you.

- **You're stuck in your ways.** After living alone for a while, you like waking up at a certain time and doing things your way without anyone interfering. Unfortunately, these habits become more ingrained with age. As we retreat further into our cocoons, we cut ourselves off from people as we stay at home, night after night, for comfort. Soon, you start to regret crawling into your pajamas so early, but it's hard to change course. It takes bravery to push yourself out of your comfort zone, but you can do it.

- **You created a set of rules that limit your choices.** Similar to the previous point, you may be tempted to follow your head rather than your heart. If you decide you want a person with a certain income level, for example, you may overlook a delightful human being who would make you feel twenty again. Or if you dated a brunette who broke your heart, you might be avoiding anyone with that hair color. You wouldn't want someone to cut you from their list for one small trait, so why limit yourself when you imagine your possible mates? Interracial relationships and same-sex relationships are far more accepted in this day and age, too, so that opens up a whole new field of candidates depending on your preferences.

- **You've lost your confidence.** Dating is hard. Let's just say it since you're probably thinking it. When you look in the mirror, you may wonder why anyone would want to spend time with you. We all have little voices that play up our fears and insecurities. Yet, you can reprogram your mind and physiology to look at your positive traits and highlight them, both in body language and conversation styles (which are covered in the chapters ahead). Without those steps, you may be sending silent signals to others that will discourage them from reaching out to you.

- **You think potential partners want someone younger or prettier.** This goes for men and women. There is often a perception that youth is more attractive, but don't discount what a person of a similar generation has to share. While some people do opt for younger partners, most people over sixty seek out someone who 'speaks their language' in terms of pop culture, cuisine, and historical references. Stop focusing on how you compare to others and predicting rejection. Instead, commit to sprucing yourself up to play up your best assets so you can shine when the right person comes along.

- **You've got heavy baggage.** By this point in your life, another person has probably hurt or neglected you, making you wary of starting over. That is only natural. However, you have the choice to be bitter and hold yourself back OR to try again for a better result. Making yourself vulnerable isn't easy, so acknowledge that feeling. It may be hard to trust other people again, especially if your scars go back to your childhood experiences or a partner who really damaged your faith in humanity. On the other hand, your next round of romance could be completely different. Believe in the brighter future that you deserve.

- **You choose the wrong 'type.'** If you've been drawn to 'bad' boys or girls in your earlier relationships, or 'safe' ones, or people who are like your parents – then figure out why you've followed that pattern. While you may have followed a particular path before, you can deviate from it this time. Clearly, your initial forays didn't work out, so break out of your mold. Think about what you could have done differently to make those connections work out better and learn from them. Then move on. If you're used to resolving disputes with fighting or the silent treatment, you will likely be happier with a partner who is calm and talks things through. It may feel foreign at first, but it may be just what you need.

- **You're afraid.** It feels safer to be alone than to venture out and be rejected, right? But don't assume the second step of that equation will happen. Fear of rejection is a deep-rooted doubt since it ties so closely to our need for emotional security. If you've been in a situation where you were 'into' someone who didn't reciprocate, it can shake your confidence. Rather than try again, you may just decide it's too much risk or opt to push someone away before they get a chance to get close. If you do that, the only person that loses out is you.

- **Your life has been busy with family commitments.** Family comes first for so many of us, particularly for the so-called 'Sandwich Generation.' We are often caring for our children who are leaving the nest later in life, while driving our parents to medical appointments. Some of us are helping out with grandchildren after our own children saw their partnerships end. At some time, you're going to have to consider your needs too. Carve out some time for you. You'll see in the pages ahead that a few minutes a day to focus on your health and happiness can really get your vision and actions realigned.

- **You're picky.** Let's just put it out there. You might want someone who is just like your former spouse or that woman you dated in college... or your brother's wonderful wife. Or the exact opposite. With dating, you cannot shop from a catalog. You will have to accept that each person you'll meet comes with a few attributes that aren't on your checklist. Rather than rejecting someone because they carry a few more pounds than you'd like, listen to the lilt of their voice or see what kind of sense of humor they have. Those are timeless traits that will enrich your life more than fitting a specific mold. The same applies to the pace of a relationship. You may want to go slowly or marry within a year. Keep your mind open to flexing your vision of a possible relationship for the long term. You may be intimidated when someone wants to see you more often than you expected. Go with it at first. See where it takes you before you start blocking their calls. You could end up very happy together.

TECHNOLOGY HAS CHANGED THE LANDSCAPE

As you have likely learned from communicating with far-flung friends, children, or grandchildren, technology has allowed us to communicate with people all around the world (or even with our neighbor down the street) without leaving our homes. If you haven't bought or been gifted an iPad or tablet yet, you may be surprised by how easy it is to dial up a friend and chat on a screen, no matter where you are.

This has changed the rules in a number of ways. For starters, you can connect with people who live in other parts of your region, country, or the world just as easily as a person on the next block. That opens up a whole new pool of possibilities as you seek out a person on your wavelength. It's now easier to track down that old flame from university or your former office to see what they are doing now.

The advent of online dating (don't cringe until we've talked about how it can work for you) has opened up countless courtships around the globe. Just meeting people from other nations can lead to wonderful conversations without having to pursue a romance.

Additionally, this also takes away the pressure to meet in person. Even if your new friend lives in the same town, you don't need to dress up to go out for a date. If you have trouble getting out of your home or driving, especially in inclement weather, you can still see each other. In times gone by, you may have just dialed each other up on the phone, but this way, you can have a face-to-face conversation, which feels more personal.

WHAT IS THE UPSIDE OF HAVING A PARTNER AT THIS POINT IN MY LIFE?

While all this technology can sound daunting, don't give up on traditional ways to meet people. It's important to remember the fun you can have dancing, laughing, or traveling with someone who makes you smile. There are many other reasons why having a healthy relationship is good for your body, mind, and social life.

People who have a close relationship are typically happier. Not only do they get to share their highs and lows with a caring listener, they actually have higher levels of naturally occurring oxytocin in the brains. Now, that's an incentive if I've ever heard of one! At the same time, you produce lower levels of cortisol – often known as the stress hormone – when you have a consistent social support buddy.

With less cortisol pumping through your system, you also sleep better. Women, in particular, feel safer with a partner sleeping beside them, leading them to doze off more quickly and rest more deeply. Combined, these effects help you cope with hardships and physical pain far better than people who are alone.

People in stable, happy relationships also have better heart health. One theory states that this could be due to people sharing their symptoms with their partner and being encouraged to seek out medical help when they need it. It's easy to dismiss the odd ache or pain, but an objective person may see patterns you don't. You may know that early intervention makes a big difference, but you may hesitate when you feel 'off' and cannot put your finger on why.

Being in a couple is also good for your mental health. Not only are you less isolated (and feel less isolated) because of the time spent with your partner, but couples also tend to socialize with other couples, so your network becomes even more extensive. You are also more likely to head to a movie or the theatre if you have a companion.

Getting out of the house and into a new setting is excellent for your brain and your mood. On the flip side, loneliness has been deemed an epidemic in the United Kingdom due to how it takes away mental stimulation and can lead to more sedentary habits and substance abuse. After all, if you are sadder and feel more alone, you are more likely to drink alcohol or pop pills to feel better.

As we age, we have more free time for relationships and to travel to all those places on our bucket list. It's more fun – and far safer – to travel with someone who can share the driving, watch your luggage in an airport, or shoot videos of you on your latest adventure. They can also suggest locales that you may not have even imagined, opening up your eyes to whole new parts of the world. Plus, you'll have more fun dressing up for dinner knowing that you'll draw a compliment from someone who cares for you and wants you to feel special.

Deep down, we all want to be loved. While our siblings and children can fill that role to some extent, having a romantic or sexual partner offers a different level of intimacy we all may crave.

For men, more so than women, having a partner to care about gives you purpose. After having a job that defined your life, you may feel adrift in retirement or in the later stages of your career. By fixing up things around the house or helping out by running errands, you feel needed. While everyone likes to be pampered by their partner, dividing up tasks allows both parties to share their skills to benefit the other person.

Of course, women who love to cook can still whip up dinners that make their partners feel special. Somehow, women seem better able to settle into a quiet retirement or find rewarding work in volunteering or meeting with friends due to a propensity to network outside of structured environments better than men.

If you've had bad experiences before, it's important to realize that, as men age, they see relationships differently. With less of a focus on sex drive, they appreciate women more for their intelligence and advice on making major life decisions. They also become more romantic as they seek deeper connections.

Humor remains a common bond at any age, regardless of gender. With maturity comes the ability to access a broader range of emotions, turning less often to the drama of your younger years. Now that you have this perspective, it's great to have a partner who has also mellowed and learned not to "sweat the small stuff." You can probably laugh more at yourself than you used to, which is a great life skill and stress reliever.

Your focus should be on finding someone who shares your values, so you don't squabble during your time together. Seek out someone who likes you for being yourself. Take the time to be choosier and the rewards will be a healthier, happier you, with someone who has settled comfortably into their own skin.

Generally, you are more likely to get out more often, try new things, and learn more if you are in a relationship. All these things enrich your days and alleviate your stress levels.

KEY TAKEAWAYS

There is a large pool of people in the same situation as you, looking for companionship for the many years of life they have ahead.

You can find someone nearby or at a distance due to technology that connects people easily, no matter where they are in the world.

Having the right partner makes you a healthier, happier person who is more likely to travel (close to home and beyond) and have more mental stimulation (and fun!).

2

WHO ARE YOU?

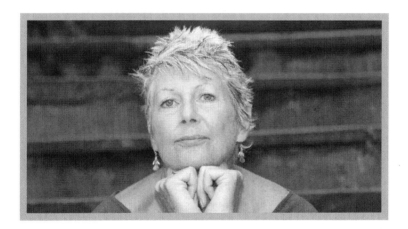

After her beloved husband died, Elaine found herself lost. As much as her children and grandchildren offered their love and support, she just couldn't have the same type of conversations with them that she used to have with Dave. She hated eating meal after meal alone, then watching TV without having someone to kibitz with over the plotlines or the sports scores. She genuinely didn't know who she was anymore, now that

she was no longer Dave's wife. Up to this point in her life, she had defined herself as the other half of a couple who went out with friends as a duo. No matter where she turned, she felt alone.

So much of our identities get caught up in what we do with our partners, especially when we become used to socializing together. In many relationships, one person cooks the meals or balances the checkbook, and it's overwhelming to take on those tasks if you haven't done them in years. After the end of any relationship, whether it's due to a death or a decision, you need to recalibrate before you can get your feet back under you again. Even if you have been single for a long time, you begin to see yourself in only one way.

In any case, you may feel rusty when it comes to dating. So how do you shake off that feeling and start anew, guilt-free?

Let's begin by examining who you are on your own. Did you quell a small part of yourself in order to function as a couple? If so, there is no reason to hold back now. Even if you had a healthy relationship, you may have given up certain habits to blend harmoniously with your partner.

If you were caring for a sick spouse, you might have had to give up your time to be home or to drive to medical appointments. That's understandable, but now you have the freedom to eat meals at different times or to return to an activity you enjoyed. That freedom can feel as scary as it does liberating since it marks a new chapter in your life.

If you've been living on your own, you face a different challenge. You've been operating on your own schedule, and you don't want to lose your independence, but you know you want to share your life in some fashion. Regardless of where you're coming from, you need to assess where you stand and what you want, before you go out looking for your match. You know what happens when you go shopping without a list. You're far more likely to pick up things you don't need and may regret later. You can easily avoid that trap by assessing what void you want to fill.

WHAT TRULY MAKES YOU HAPPY?

"It takes courage to grow up and become who you really are."
– E. E. Cummings

After years of living up to the expectations of your boss, partner, or the needs of your kids, it can be challenging to let go of your identity as an employee, spouse, or another defining role. You may have lost sight of your true self. This is especially hard if you have just retired, lost your job, or your kids have moved out of your home. This is truly a time to start your next chapter.

Imagine you're at a cocktail party and someone asks you, "What do you do?". If you fall into the default response of listing your job or number of children, is that your true personality? In a minute or less, you have created your first impression with another person. Did you make the most of it? I love when I get a conversation-opening response about a person's passion – whether it's an artistic project, an exotic voyage, or an exciting hobby that raises so many more questions. Don't you want that to be you? Life tries to slot us into tidy spaces, but we don't have to follow the rules. In order to craft an answer that will leave you smiling, you have to look deeply into yourself and enjoy the journey.

Open up by thinking about the five to ten moments in your life that brought you true joy. Weddings and the birth of children don't count, since those milestones are often universal. Write down the list. Next, ponder each one and why it sticks out for you. Dig into the emotions that came with it and the reaction you received, both internally and externally. Depending if you are a verbal or written communicator, you can either find a sounding board to discuss these highlights or scrawl down the words that jump to mind as you revisit them. Revel in the memories as you laugh and smile. Don't you want to feel that joy more often? To do so, you need to go to the core of the reason why they stand out for you.

Maybe they tapped you as a mentor, a cheerleader, or an advocate? Did they allow you to try something new or learn a new skill? How far did they take you beyond your comfort zone, if at all? They may have helped you reach a goal, solve a problem, or overcome a challenge. Whatever it was, each one sparked your spirit and spoke to who you truly are. Follow that compass point as you ask yourself more illuminating questions.

What would you do if you could do anything? Forget about money or what anyone else would think. Some people would jump on a plane and travel to a destination they have had in their hearts for years. Others would do home renovations to make their home a greater place of pride and comfort. A retired teacher could find a volunteer role as a literacy coach. A person who gave up their motorcycle license years ago may go out and renew it. A dissatisfied employee could finally quit that toxic job and find one with more meaning.

Just thinking about your own options gets your juices flowing. You don't have to go in full tilt, but you just showed yourself another glimpse of your passions, desires, and possibilities. Even if you only go one step towards that goal, you are that much closer.

Picture yourself winning the lottery. Would you stay in your current home? How much of your wealth would you share? What treats would you give yourself? Again, this isn't about money, but freeing yourself up to dream about your long-term future. You have already looked at what sparked your joy in the past and considered what steps you would take in the near future if your parameters were not limited. Now, look further into the horizon.

We always assume winning big would lead to happiness, but often the idea of coming into unexpected cash is more fun than the reality of it. Just in case your numbers are coming up soon, you might as well plan for it! This is your life. Make the best of it by not just focusing on past highlights, but ensuring some of your best moments are yet to come.

Now, next time someone asks you, "What do you do?" you should have a great answer ready.

WHAT ARE YOUR CORE VALUES?

Most of us have not looked deeply inside our authentic selves to ask what we need. You grew up, went to school, got a job, and maybe met the love of your life... then lost them. Starting over wasn't part of your plan – until now. However, it's a great time to ask yourself what is important to you, so you can find what you're really seeking in a relationship.

The best couples always seem to be on the same wavelength. You've seen the people who take trips together and come back raving about how much fun they had. Likewise, duos who like to dine out with gusto clearly agree on the type of food they like, and both enjoy splurging on restaurant meals. However, if they don't share the same values, then there will be conflict.

For Elaine and Dave, eating out was a rare luxury for special occasions. Instead, she loved batch cooking meals and having intimate dinners at home where they reviewed the highs and lows of their days. Although Dave didn't live long enough to get there, they saved up a nice little nest egg for their retirement years. Now, she has money set aside and no one to share it with. And she couldn't decide what to do with it since she had always discussed financial matters with her husband.

If you're feeling a little murky about your values, you may automatically say your family or your health is your top priority. Those are easy, go-to statements that don't really go below the surface. However, we are all complex beings who interpret the world in so many ways. If you turn to any online values assessments, you will see lists of values that you can choose from to summarize how you really think and function.

For example, the Barrett Values Centre asks you to choose ten values out of a long list and emails you a report. It assesses where you stand on a scale from basic survival mode to the need for a loving and protective relationship, good self-esteem, the process of letting go for transformation, a focus on meaning in existence, the desire to make a difference in the world, and selfless service. It builds on Maslow's Hierarchy of Needs, which has five levels: physiological needs, safety, love and belonging, esteem, and self-actualization. There are various free and paid value-assessing options, depending on how deep you wish to go. The one hosted by Psychology Today takes almost an hour and costs $7, giving you a rich analysis.

In general, these assessments open up the process so you can look at several aspects of your life, such as:

- Do you need to be in control of your time and finances, or are you willing to be flexible?
- Do you have to have your home orderly and clean at all times?
- Do you like to spend your time with small groups or go out at every opportunity?

- Is volunteering vital to your sense of self-worth?
- Where do you spend your money – travel, feathering your nest, saving for the future, or buying flattering clothes so you look sharp?
- Are you a planner with a structured schedule, or do you go with whatever is happening at the moment?
- Are truth and personal ethics important to you?
- Are you playful, or do you prefer being a grown-up who takes life seriously?
- Do you need the constant stimulation of the radio or TV, or do you thrive in silence?
- Is your faith central to your life?
- Are you constantly learning, or do you just want to relax and turn to your regular comforts of reruns and beloved books?

All these questions – and more like them – give you a sense of what is important to you. There are no right or wrong answers. You need to be true to yourself, so you know what you want to stand up for when someone asks you to bend a little. This is a beautiful chance for you to look inside yourself as an individual rather than as half of a couple. Don't settle for someone else's image of you. Write your own list and keep it handy. It's actually really liberating.

Celebrate the great things about precious *you*. Do you have infectious energy? A bright smile? Fun dance moves? A kind heart? A killer sense of humor? Brilliant baking skills? Every person has a series of gifts they bring to the table, and you are no different. You just need to tap into what makes you unique and bring it to the forefront of your mind. That way, it will be harder to resist your charms.

For Elaine, she discovered that she liked the traditions that she and Dave had created, with one exception. She liked treating herself to the occasional lunch out with friends to try new dishes. That meant she didn't eat alone as often, and she justified the expense by going to mid-range restaurants and not dining out on the more expensive dinner menu. She was surprised how much she enjoyed this treat of dressing up and going out a few days a week.

* * *

WEEK 1 ASSIGNMENTS

❖ Take a few pictures of yourself, including a headshot and an image of your entire body clothed. If you're not used to being on this end of the lens, don't be shy. Just do it so we can compare your photo now to one that you will take at the end of the twelve-week program.

❖ Sit down and brainstorm all the words that describe who you are. The values exercise may help you get started, but let's build on it. Seek out neutral or positive words, such as friendly, heart-centered, chatty, trustworthy, etc. Write them in your journal. This will not be a definitive list. You will build on it as we go through each week.

KEY TAKEAWAYS

By taking a good, hard look at who you are, you get a better understanding of yourself and your needs at this point in your life.

Consider which parts of your life are the most important to you, so you stick with those values as you meet new people.

3

LET GO OF PAST HEARTACHE TO BEGIN ANEW

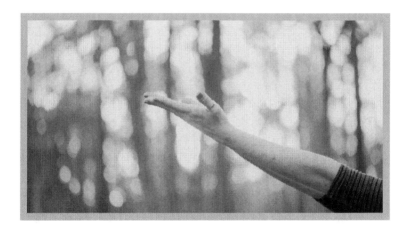

*E*very relationship in our lives leaves a little residue behind, whether it's a fond memory or a lesson learned. When it comes to romance or companionship, it may be hard to release the parts that we loved or that have damaged our hearts. It's hard to move on until you have given yourself permission to do so. This is rarely easy since it is such an emotional step. If you have loved someone deeply, you will never stop grieving their disappearance from your life.

When do you know you are ready for this step? After all, there is no schedule that you need to follow. Some people marry within a year of the death of their spouse when the right person comes along. Some relationship 'experts' say it takes up to three years before your heart has mended sufficiently to allow someone else into it. While you often hear about having a quick, rebound relationship to get someone out of your system, I wouldn't recommend this type of approach. It's not fair to the other person, who may be seeking a deeper relationship. Instead, take the time you need. Only you will know when you're ready to open yourself up again.

There are clear signs of when you have reached that point:

- When you lose someone – to divorce, a
  relocation, or a death – they will probably linger
  in your thoughts for a long time. You may feel
  that they may call, or you can feel their presence
  in your daily life. It's hard when another person is
  so ingrained in your habits and your heart.
  However, one day, you may find that they haven't
  crossed your mind in hours. If that person has
  died, you may feel guilty about not hanging onto
  those memories. However, you will always have a
  piece of them in your heart. You are still living,
  and you need to be happy again. If that person
  truly loved you in return, they would likely want
  you to find peace and joy as well. Don't fight it.

But do watch for it and acknowledge it when it happens.

- At the same time, you may find that you cannot talk about a loved one without tears springing to your eyes. If someone has hurt you, you will carry the scars for a while. Often, triggers make you think of them, such as a specific aroma, a song, or even an expression the person used regularly. If you are a widow or widower, you have reached a key milestone if you can laugh or smile without falling into grief. For turbulent relationships, being able to cope with a trigger without hearing a critical voice in your head is a good turning point for you. Embrace it and get ready to open up your heart again.

- Some people rehash their breakups often, trying to understand what went wrong and why. You may not even realize how earnestly you're doing it. Try to be more aware of how often you refer to your ex and ask yourself why you're still talking about him or her. You can invite friends to track this as well and remind you that you're falling into this habit. If you are still checking their social media feeds, you have to ask yourself why. Keeping this flame burning isn't doing you any good. If you need to, symbolically burn or toss out certain mementos that keep you connected.

Once you can get past this phase, the more open you will be to new possibilities. Only then can you ask yourself the following key question.

WHAT KIND OF PARTNER DO YOU WANT?

Ask yourself honestly if you want to end up in the same type of relationship you had before or if you want something different. Some people long to have the perceived security of marriage, while others prefer to live independently and see their partner periodically. If you like having company for dinner and a companion at concerts, you don't need to marry and have that person sharing your living space.

Just as with the values question, there is no right or wrong way to live your life. It's yours, so it's best to be honest with yourself about what you need right now. The options could be a spouse, common-law partner, companion, lover, travel buddy, or a friend for social outings.

Based on what you've assessed about yourself and your life at this point, what do you feel is missing? You obviously picked up this book for a reason. You're feeling ready to step into something new, so now you should define what would be the ultimate goal for you. Take a look at where you feel the gaps most keenly and write down what would be the ideal arrangement for you.

After living with a previous partner, you may yearn for the same day-to-day partnership, or you might relish your newfound freedom and not want to give it up. If you have always lived a single life, you can create boundaries around what you're willing to share and what space you need on your own. That's okay.

If all goes as planned, one day a wonderful person will ask you what you want out of a relationship, so it's best to have an answer formulated. That way, you will not feel pressured to give in to whatever the other person wants. At your age, you can stand up for what you believe and get the type of alliance you want. Of course, you can always change your mind if the chemistry with the right person inspires you. You can write your own rules and adapt them as you get back into the dating game.

Once you have set your sights on who you are and what you are aiming to change, you can focus on the exact type of person who fits the bill without getting your heart broken unnecessarily (or breaking theirs). Ultimately, you want to make decisions that focus you, so when we go through subsequent chapters, you can easily choose activities and the appropriate settings to seek out the right companion for you. Follow your heart and you cannot go wrong.

* * *

WEEK 2 ASSIGNMENTS

❖ By now, you've got a great start to your list of positive attributes about yourself, so keep going. Now that you know what you want, you can think about words that fit that model. For example, you may feel you are loyal or free-spirited. As long as you are honest, that's what matters.

❖ Next, write a short letter about a past relationship. This letter is for your eyes only. If your ex is still around, do not mail it or share anything about it on social media. Simply say 'thank you' for the past experience and all the learning, but you acknowledge that you are now moving on. If your partner has passed away, write a short letter (if you can) about how much you miss them and reassure them that you are continuing your life in a positive way while deciding to attract new people into your life. If you can't write the words, then say them out loud in a heartfelt way. Whichever situation you are in, tell that person how you have great optimism that your life will only be better from this point forward.

KEY TAKEAWAYS

You cannot move into a healthy relationship until you let go of the one(s) left behind. Physically say goodbye so you can move on in a positive way.

Ask yourself what you need in your life right now and set out to fill that gap. This is an individual decision, so look into your heart and do what is right for you.

4

UPGRADED YOU

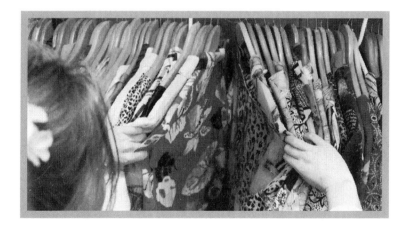

*N*ow that you've done a self-assessment of your wonderful inner self – and have documented it with a smile – it's time to look at the way you present yourself to the world. If you've been living for 'comfort only' for months, take a moment or two to consider your appearance and your surroundings. You don't need a total makeover, but maybe a little spruce-up so you feel a little younger physically, mentally, and emotionally. This isn't really for others. It's another way to refresh your mindset, and as a bonus, you'll look a little more stylish to the world.

By refreshing your surroundings, your outfits, and your body, you will infuse yourself with renewed energy that will be infectious. Just try it and see how much it brightens up your life.

DECLUTTER YOUR HOUSE (AND YOUR MIND)

Just as you let go of your past relationships by saying goodbye, now you need to do the same with the stuff around you. Face it, you cannot get a fresh start if your environment is littered with too many pieces of your past life. I'm not saying you should toss your photo albums, but you may be hanging onto things for the wrong reasons. This is an excellent time to declutter your home, starting with a spare bedroom closet or junk drawer. We always feel good when we do spring cleaning since it clears our minds too. Once you've tackled that task, you can take on a larger challenge.

Begin the second step by looking at your wardrobe and tossing things from your past. Yes, you loved that sweater, but after thirty years, it's likely showing wear and tear. Did you buy something luxurious then lose the nerve to wear it? Ladies, are you hanging onto bras you purchased for that backless dress for your sister's wedding thirty years ago? Gentlemen, how many pairs of your underwear have holes in them? Let's take another look at every item you own and decide if it belongs in your life or not.

Automatically, get rid of anything that is five years old or older, unless it is a timeless classic. If you've had something since pre-1980, kiss it goodbye, since those trends are never coming back, especially for a mature adult. Ditto for anything that doesn't fit or is unflattering. Why waste space on something that doesn't make you shine?

We typically own far more clothing than we can ever wear. Unless you only do laundry once a month, the average person can get by with two suits, a nice pair of dress pants, a few fitted cotton shirts, a few sweaters, a nice coat, a pencil skirt (for women), and shoes for going out, working out and dressing up.

With these guidelines in mind, tackle each closet, dresser, and trunk and separate everything into five piles: toss (for anything worn out or stained), mend (for that shirt that is just missing a button or has a torn seam), sell (for quality items that just aren't *you* anymore), share (with a friend or relative), and store. The final pile is for sentimental items that you just cannot discard, but set the bar high. Keep the suit or dress from life-defining moments only.

I recommend physically dumping everything on a bed or table and only returning vital, flattering items to your closet or drawers. Once you do this, you will be amazed at the space you have and how much easier it is to find what you need and want to wear. It's a nice reset. If you've thinned out more than you expected, then treat yourself to a shopping spree to pick up the exact items you need –

and nothing more. Make sure the colors and textures bring you joy.

Next, slip on something that makes you feel fabulous or dashing and stand in front of the mirror. Take a good look at your hair, nails, and shoes. Is your underwear droopy or offering less support than you need? Your next outing could be to the store to get some nice new silky or slimming undergarments. If your hairstyle doesn't meet your expectations, set up an appointment for a trim, color, or whatever service you feel you need. Invest in yourself for your own sake, before you even think of trying to please anyone else. It will really perk up your spirits and your confidence.

MOVE THOSE MUSCLES

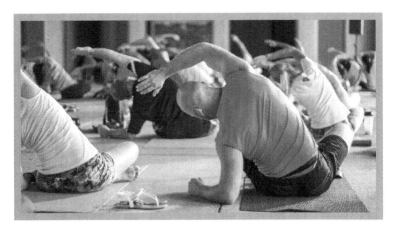

As we get older, we typically move less. By the time most adults turn seventy-five, only two-thirds of men and half of women still exercise regularly. Yet, the benefits of keeping active are incredible. Regular exercise lowers your risk for heart disease, high blood pressure, diabetes, arthritis, and various cancers and makes you more flexible, strong, resilient, and capable of living independently for longer. By working on your balance, you can train your body to prevent you from falling and injuring yourself, especially if your bones aren't as strong as they used to be.[4] And you'll have more energy that you can use to participate in fun activities. In case you hadn't noticed, fit people tend to be more confident and willing to try new things. That's another motivator right there.

That doesn't mean you need to rush out and sign up for a kickboxing class. Ideally, you'll want to focus on some type of movement to get stronger and improve your balance and posture. It doesn't have to be strenuous either; the trick is to do it daily, so you get the perks by building on what you've done the previous day. If you haven't been active for a while, get out for a walk and enjoy the scenery. Getting outside also lifts your mood and offers a refreshing change of setting. Start with just five minutes at first to see how it feels, then go for as long as it feels comfortable to do so.

After you've been walking for a few days, pick up the pace a little or tackle a flight of stairs to get your heart pumping a little bit more. Don't overdo it since that will only set you back. Ramp up slowly, so you don't pull a muscle and fall out of the habit before you really settle into it. Rather than seeing this as a chore, look at it as time indulging yourself in a natural action that gets your endorphins rolling.

You can also build up your stamina by doing yard work or cleaning your house, but that should be in addition to a regular workout. Add some small weights to strengthen your upper body and your bones. Again, never overdo it since it takes longer to heal from muscle strains once you're over the age of sixty.

If you prefer a scheduled activity to keep you disciplined, sign up for a yoga class or learn how to do Pilates or tai chi. All of these gentle exercise programs make your core and legs stronger while limbering up your joints. Who knows? You may meet a new friend – of the same sex or not – who expands your social network. Either way, you'll get a glow that others won't be able to ignore.

WEEK 3 ASSIGNMENTS

You didn't think I forgot about your homework, did you? Here are your assignments for this week, which you can easily fit into your active days:

❖ Choose one room or closet to declutter this week. Specify which day and time you will tackle it, so you don't procrastinate. Once you get going, I'll bet you find it invigorating and keep on going. It's truly amazing what we keep around when we don't have our radar attuned to this task.

❖ Find some form of movement, such as walking, hitting the treadmill, doing yoga, stretching, or strength training, that you will perform twenty to thirty minutes a day. Start slow and enjoy the feeling of your body getting stronger and more limber each day. If you need to, schedule it as well.

❖ Continue adding positive words to describe yourself in your journal. Keep looking for ways to celebrate your good traits, so you are reminded of just how precious you are. It's okay if you accidentally repeat some words. That just makes you doubly awesome!

KEY TAKEAWAYS

By clearing out old clothes and other clutter, you focus on what you need and want, which also hones your mindset for your future search for love or companionship.

Getting your body moving helps you stay healthy so you can do more in life, and maybe even shave off a few pounds.

5

REFRESH YOUR MINDSET

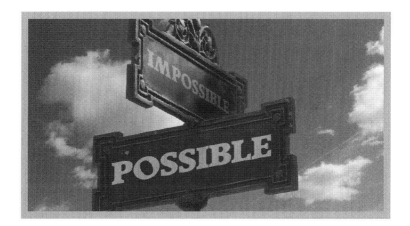

*A*s we change the physical world around us, our outlook begins to evolve as well. If we train our brains to be more optimistic, open, and nimble, we can improve our moods and stave off depression, anxiety, and even lower your risk of dementia. If that's not a motivator, then I don't know what is. This begins with how we talk to ourselves about ourselves. What words do we agree to accept from other people when they speak to us?

SEEK OUT KINDNESS

It's easy to be critical and make our tiny flaws out to be greater than they are. By being kind to yourself, you also become less tolerant of other people who are not nice to you. You don't need them and their negativity. Too often, we hang onto the critical things people say to us, but that is counterproductive. Maybe that person was just having a bad day. Don't allow them to leave a stain on your psyche.

Instead, focus on the good things you do that remind you that you are a good person. Remember the favors you've done for people, the compliments you've paid to coworkers, or the donations you've made to charities. You helped out a neighbor or volunteered for a good cause. Those are the moments that should shine above the rest, since they reflect decisions you made to make another person's day better. Those small kindnesses add up.

If you haven't had a chance to do any of these things recently, commit to doing them in the coming days. You can add your record of these deeds to a page across from where you are recording your positive traits. Soon, you will be looking for ways to build that list, since each entry you record makes you feel like you are providing the type of support to others that also brightens your days. You are on a path towards happiness and fulfillment. Spread that sunshine on the path ahead of you.

READ TO FEED YOUR BRAIN

Likewise, treat yourself to books that uplift you and teach you about topics that stimulate your brain. That way, you will seek out words and messages that reinforce your current state of mind. The most successful business leaders in the world prescribe themselves time to read and reflect each day. Again, this isn't about focusing on material wealth, but the wealth that knowledge adds to your quality of life. Even if you didn't enjoy reading earlier in life, you can now opt for titles that speak to your interests without having deadlines or other pressures that make it a chore.

Investor extraordinaire Warren Buffett committed to reading at least 500 pages every day and often exceeded that target. Philanthropist and tech giant Bill Gates tears through one book each week.[5] While you don't need to push yourself to that pace, challenge yourself to one or two per month at first and see how much you enjoy meeting new characters and influential people on the written page.

A lifelong learner has a curious and nimble mind that makes it easier for them to carry on sparkling conversations. Joining this club is as easy as heading to your nearest library or bookstore. You can also exchange books with friends, which gets you out socializing as well. As you pick books off the shelves, aim to choose enriching and enlightening material to suit your goals ahead. Sure, you can work in some romance, drama, and mystery. Now, imagine introducing yourself at cocktail parties as an avid reader and let the repartee carry on from there!

BE GRATEFUL

As we go through our day-to-day life, it's easy to talk about the jerk that cut you off in traffic or the shopper who was rude to you at the supermarket. However, I am going to challenge you to look at the other side of the equation and try to look at the world with fresh eyes. Aren't you lucky to afford a car to run your errands, and isn't it grand that you have enough money to buy food? See, now you're looking at the glass like it's half full – or hopefully more.

Finding gratitude actually rewires our brains to deal with stress and toxic emotions better. A University of California, Berkeley study showed that people who wrote thank-you letters, whether they mailed them or not, had more activity in their prefrontal cortex.[6] This part of the frontal lobe regulates how we respond to information and which feelings we use when making decisions. In other words, it makes us wiser.

Every day, something good happens to you. You just have to look for the small graces that bless you. You get out of bed and stand up under your own power. You live in a safe home. Savor every moment as you eat fresh food, stand under the stream of a warm shower, or talk with a caring friend or family member.

WRITE DOWN YOUR POSITIVE THOUGHTS

Start banking those joyful moments and recording them so you can remind yourself how lucky you are. Sometimes, it may be tough to find a bright spot. When that happens, flip back to your list of good times and take steps to cheer up. That may mean you have to pick up the phone and call your sister or take yourself out in the sunshine for a recharge.

If your words don't inspire you enough, you can always use quotes and affirmations from other writers to start each day on the right foot. Consider these gems:

"I awoke this morning with devout thanksgiving for my friends, the old and the new."
– Ralph Waldo Emerson

* * *

"Appreciation is a wonderful thing.
It makes what is excellent in others belong to us as well."
– Voltaire

* * *

"When you arise in the morning, give thanks for the food and for the joy of living. If you see no reason for giving thanks, the fault lies only in yourself."
– Tecumseh

* * *

"Gratitude turns what we have into enough, and more. It turns denial into acceptance, chaos into order, confusion into clarity... it makes sense of our past, brings peace for today, and creates a vision for tomorrow."
– Melody Beattie

If you want to pick one up and treat yourself to a daily dose of goodness, there are entire books of quotes from inspiring entrepreneurs, moms, dads, athletes, and people from all walks of life. What reaches our brains has a considerable impact on our moods and our physical health, so keep feeding your soul positive vibes, and soon you'll be cheering up that cranky customer at Costco rather than muttering about their misbehavior. Then you will become even more delightful for others to spend time with.

TRY SOMETHING NEW

Now that you've ramped up your energy and are feeling better dressed and more empowered, you may feel up to broadening your horizons. If you've been in the same pattern for a while, adding a new activity will fire up your brain and shake up your muscle memory. Being open to novel experiences can feel scary at first, which is why we're starting small.

Now, don't limit yourself to what you 'should' do. Just because your bossy brother-in-law wants you to join his golf foursome doesn't mean you have to go along with him. Sure, you can try it out, but if it doesn't suit you, then find another way to spend your time. We still feel peer pressure at any age, but you have invested energy in looking at your needs, so don't put them second to someone else's whims.

Ideally, you want to find something that sparks joy and challenges you intellectually. Depending on your desires, you can have something scheduled, such as a weekly card game or volunteer role. You can also opt for an activity you can do on your own at any point in the day.

Here are some options to get your internal gears moving:

- Dig into your genealogy to find out where your roots began. Sites like Ancestry.com make it easy to begin the search for people from the past. You never know what – or who – you may discover!

- Why not capture your own story by writing a memoir for your children and other relatives to enjoy? While we all share stories at family gatherings, it's nice to have a thorough version on paper for future generations. You could stir up some great memories from your younger years and provide your nieces and nephews with some laughs or insights from times gone by.

- Crafts, like woodworking or quilting, not only create items that make you proud, they also call on your problem-solving skills as you work through each stage of a project.

- Pick up your camera and go exploring. Nature and architecture offer so many colors and shapes that you can capture at various angles to make your view unique. Think of different ways to present a scene to make it truly yours. And who can get enough pictures of the children in their life? Snap a few of those as well.

- Games and puzzles keep your mind agile and help reduce your risk of dementia. Pick up a crossword or Sudoku book and try to complete each page.

- Nurturing a garden does more than produce greens and flowers. People get hooked on the stimulation of picking out each plant and learning what makes it thrive. You exercise by planting and weeding while developing more patience and an appreciation for nature.

- Share the bounty of your kitchen by inviting friends in for dinners, so you're not dining alone. You can rotate the routine by dining out at their homes as well, giving you the chance to try new recipes and taste new flavors. We tend to put more love and effort into the dishes we make for others, but we can still enjoy them ourselves.

- Find out what all the fuss is about Fortnite. This popular video game and others change scenarios and levels of difficulty to keep you adapting as you play. You can take a magical journey, solve a puzzle, or participate in a race against other players while fine-tuning your reflexes and neural pathways. Playing thirty to forty-five minutes per day can improve your memory.

All these activities make you feel more alive, and they also provide a topic of conversation when you do get out to meet new people. Talk about a win-win situation!

WEEK 4 ASSIGNMENTS

❖ Carry on with the tasks from Weeks 1 to 3. Keep documenting your attributes, sorting through the detritus of your life, and exercising your body.

❖ Add in the kind deeds you did for others and the books you read as you peel through your notes. Looking back on this list (and the one above) should make you feel like you are shedding your own skin, so a new one shines through.

❖ Choose one or two inspirational quotes, or one or two inspirational affirmations that you will write out and place on your bathroom wall, in your office, or on the fridge, as a daily reminder of what is important in your life.

KEY TAKEAWAYS

Being grateful for what you have in life and drawing inspiration from others helps you stay positive and to look forward, powered by the good memories in the present.

Trying new experiences opens your mind and makes you a better conversationalist, a skill you will need very soon.

6

WHO ARE THEY?

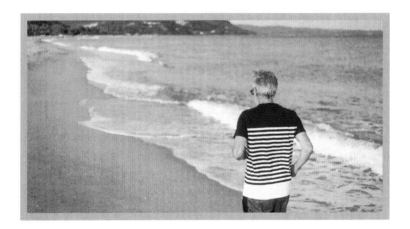

*O*nce you've got a healthy grip on who you are and what you want in a relationship, you can extend your gaze out into the world to see who will match your core values and the type of partnership that works for you. This is not a quick one-and-done exercise, since there are several things you need to keep in mind to get what you want and deserve.

After opening yourself up to new experiences and hobbies, the next logical step is to think about having a new person to enjoy them with, or even leveraging them as an icebreaker when you meet a new person. However, you don't want to lose momentum on a false start with the first person who crosses your path. So be patient and shop around for someone who truly enriches your life in the areas where you really feel there's a gap.

Nathan had married in his early twenties to his steady girlfriend of two years, mainly because that was what you did in those days. Even in the early years of their union, they had both felt they had made the wrong choice, but soldiered on for more than twenty years before they both admitted they were miserable and parted ways.

Their marriage had been a traditional one, with him relying on Kathy to prepare meals and care for their home. Soon, he found himself eating canned soup and takeout dinners that made him feel even more sluggish and out of shape. He longed for the companionship he thought he would get when he dreamt of married life on the eve of his wedding: intimate dinners where he shared the highlights and lowlights of his day, followed by discussions of where life would take them next. More than anything, he wanted the intimacy of good conversation over dessert or while drifting off to sleep at night beside someone he trusted. In return, he would happily provide economic security and loyalty, which was one of his innate characteristics. However, were there women seeking this type of old-school partnership anymore? He wasn't sure if that was a thing of the past or not.

Like Nathan, you may see precisely how you want your future life to shape up. You don't need to be constricted by what you have lived before; relationships have evolved to have a broader menu of choices from which you can choose what suits you best. As we discussed earlier, once you get clear sights on what exactly you are looking for in a potential mate, you can seek out a friend, a travel partner, a lover, a live-in partner, or a spouse.

Later-life partnerships are no longer confined to the boundaries of marriage. Older adults are taking advantage of the flexibility they can have within unmarried partnerships, including cohabitation. A growing number of people do not feel compelled to socialize only as a couple, and neither should you. If there are differences between you in terms of income, class, or other expectations[7] that could cause a strain on a partnership, you can always find ways to enjoy time together without forcing your union past a breaking point. Long-term marriages are increasingly ending in divorce, and most individuals who call it quits are not repartnering.[8]

There are several factors to consider, including your need for emotional or economic security, your health, and your vision for the next chapter of your life. All of these – and more – are invaluable to your happiness, so don't feel you need to fit into a specific mold to please anyone else.

Some widows and widowers want to marry again, while others prefer to keep their independence after years of living in close quarters. You may want to keep things casual or just find someone to travel with, whether it's on day trips or cruises to other parts of the world. It's okay if you don't want a traditional relationship.

This is your life, and you can absolutely live it your way without having to justify it to anyone. You just need to be fair with people you meet so they understand where they may fit into the vision you have. Honesty is always best, as you have likely learned by now. Having these conversations now can save you from heartache later, and I have some advice on how to navigate those potentially difficult discussions with dignity and respect.

The choice is up to you. Along the way, you may change your mind, but let's start out by seeing how you arrive at that choice in the first place. Let's go over the limitations that may be unconsciously lurking in your mind. By this point in your life, you've likely had some good and bad experiences that have shaped how you think about new relationships. If you and other family members have been abandoned or used, you may find yourself muttering stereotypes, such as "There are no men you can trust" or "All women are gold diggers." Logically, this makes no sense, but people do fall into this trap.

This is thanks to the Reticular Activating System (RAS) that lives in your brain, just at the top of your spinal column. Essentially, it tells us to focus on what our brain shows us. This network of neurons takes signals from all our senses, even our gut, and synthesizes the findings to affect our behavior. It keeps us awake and helps us to focus on the tasks we perform in our day-to-day lives, acting as a gatekeeper of information that flows in and out of our thoughts. Therefore, if it has only seen relationships lead to heartache, it hasn't 'seen' or felt what a loving rapport can add to your life. No wonder you're skittish if you've only had one or a few significant partnerships, and they haven't ended well. That's all you have known.

In another example, the RAS is behind the reflex that makes you notice a certain type of car as soon as you buy one of the same model. What is familiar to you becomes more accentuated than the other data that come to you in a day. Sure, there are dozens of other kinds of cars on the road, but they just go by unnoticed because the RAS is not pointing them out to you. The same could be said of potential partners if you're not looking for someone like them. In order to remove your blinders, you need to retrain your brain not to automatically react only to the things and experiences you are accustomed to experiencing.

This begins by looking at yourself differently, then designing the life you want, rather than the one you have. It's like eating the same junk food and knowing you won't lose weight, or staying in a job that constrains you knowing that you have to apply elsewhere to get a fresh start. It can feel daunting to venture into new waters, but it's much easier when you realize you're not in a healthy place to begin with. This change in thinking and beliefs doesn't come naturally, so try to become aware of your limiting thoughts so they don't hold you back. Journaling about the life ahead can pave the way for a smoother transition.

As self-development author Brian Tracey wisely says, "The key to success is to focus our conscious mind on things we desire, not things we fear."

RANKING YOUR NEEDS, WANTS, AND DEAL-BREAKERS

While you may have an ideal situation or person in mind, you need to draw the lines between what is carved in stone, scrawled in ink, and sketched in pencil as you go forward. It would be lovely if you found someone who checks ALL your boxes, but it's also helpful to understand what traits and habits are vital and which ones are only 'nice to have.' Some choices will be obvious, but others may pop up as you consider other people's relationships or even watch TV shows where couples interact.

Get out a piece of paper and divide it into three columns. Start drafting lists of what you want to make your relationship perfect, what you need to feel safe and loved, and what deal-breakers are non-negotiable.

For example:

- Some people can make long-distance relationships work, since both partners enjoy having their independence. However, if you want in-person companionship daily or several times a week, you must have someone who lives within a short driving distance of your home.

- If you cannot stand the smell of tobacco smoke, then you obviously will struggle to become physically close to a smoker. Perhaps it dredges up old memories of a toxic environment, or you lost a loved one to emphysema and don't want to go through that pain again. Put it on the list.

- Anyone who has survived an abusive relationship – whether you're male or female – will need to live within specific rules about conflict resolution and critical language. If you end up with someone who makes you feel small or under-appreciated, that's a no-go right from the start.

On the upside, you can have some fun imagining what you can do with a new partner and how they will make you feel. Just imagining yourself in this situation gets your hopeful hormones rolling, and you can see beyond the limits of your Reticular Activating System's experiences so far.

The first draft of Nathan's initial list looked something like this (to get you started, there is a blank grid in the appendix, but you can write down some early thoughts on any piece of paper available):

Wants	Needs	Deal-Breakers
Someone fun	Cooking skills (to teach me)	Live close by
Ages 60-67	Independent driver	Non-smoker
Shared interest in history	Interest in traveling	Good conversationalist
Movie buff	Financially astute	Willing to do things as a couple

After considering the life he aimed to share, he decided he **wanted** someone fun who took things less seriously than Kathy had when they were together. He also chose a range of ages he thought would be suitable, but was open to someone slightly older or a little younger. While he hoped his new friend would share some of his interests, he was also open to learning about hers.

For the next column, he felt he **needed** someone who could cook beyond his basic skills to provide him a sense of comfort and better nutrition, even if she could just teach him how to prepare better meals for himself. After driving his wife around for years, since she never wanted to get her license, he needed someone to share the time behind the wheel, especially if he started to take all the road trips Kathy had refused to join in with. He was also wary of taking on another person's debts after living judiciously on a single income for so many years.

As for **deal-breakers**, he wanted someone in his life regularly – preferably daily – but was vehemently anti-smoking. Most of all, he couldn't end up in a quiet house with a silent partner again since he really wanted the camaraderie that good matches share when they explore the world together then rehash the memories in vivid detail. His parents and siblings had those types of rapport, and he realized how jealous he had been of them all these years. (Spoiler alert: He found her while volunteering and has been enjoying her Italian home cooking and zest for international travel ever since. They are divinely happy together as he also became a stepfather and a grandfather, milestones he never thought he would achieve.)

Like Nathan, you will be figuring out what components make up this person who complements you, not completes you. You are still wonderful you – with a side-kick who makes you even better. While you may share some interests, having someone who has stronger skills in the kitchen or with finances can take the pressure off a partner who finds that part of life less fulfilling. Like musicians who play well together, you aim to make beautiful music by harmonizing your lives and bringing out the best in each other – whoever that other person will be...

* * *

WEEK 5 ASSIGNMENTS

❖ Carry on with the tasks from Weeks 1 to 4. Keep writing down your good points, trying new activities, and tackling one more closet or drawer to toss out clutter.

❖ As more inspirational quotes and affirmations come into view (this is where your Reticular Activating System comes in handy), put them up around your home to keep your spirits up and your mind planning for brighter days ahead.

❖ Draft your list of wants, needs, and deal-breakers without capping it off. More ideas will pop up as we work through the next steps. Keep an open mind at all times.

KEY TAKEAWAYS

Every person has their own version of the mate they want, from interests to expectations in a relationship. No two people have the same list, so don't give in to peer pressure.

Listen for the voices in your head that limit your choices or discourage you from finding a new partner. Recognize them, but reach further to truly find happiness.

Creating a hierarchy of what you want, need, and must have (or the inverse) will come in handy as you meet and vet people in the coming weeks and months.

7

GET SOCIAL – PRACTICE YOUR SKILLS

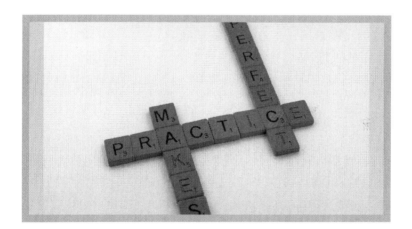

$\mathcal{O}$nce you decide to get out and meet new people, you may need a refresher on how to flirt or even start a conversation with someone new. If you're rusty, it may take some practice before this feels natural again, but your newfound confidence and your recent round of decisions should help you feel more grounded. Breaking the ice with new people can be intimidating for those of us who are shyer. However, when you think back on all the challenges you've faced in your life, you should be able to shake off your reticence and feel ready to make the first move. As with any other habit, you start with small steps and build up your nerve with conversations that feel less risky and emotionally invested.

After being cooped up for a while or out of the dating mix for a few years, it can feel strange to get out and about with other people, especially if you have established a comfortable routine or have kept your social network tight-knit. However, it is healthy to leave your nest for brief periods at first, get involved with activities beyond your home, and practice being social again. So, if you doubt you're up to it, take a deep breath. Think of it like riding a bike and believe that you can do it again.

Like any other skill, you get better at it when you practice, practice, practice. Remember those piano lessons, after-noons at the driving range, hours at the rink – or whatever activity kept you busy when you were younger? This is just like that. After a few potentially awkward starts, you will find your groove, and it will feel more natural to interact with people you haven't met before. You can do this!

Begin with some easy conversations. Perhaps you see your mail carrier daily but linger inside until your letters are in your box. Instead, pop out and wish this person a cheery hello. Strike up short discussions with people in elevators when you're between floors to break up the silence, commenting on the weather, or delivering a compliment.

Get out of your car when you go to buy a coffee and start talking with other people in line. You will see more opportunities to brighten other people's day, whether you're buying groceries or picking up a parcel at the post office.

The more you ask questions or share small talk, the easier it gets. While it may seem intrusive at first, you may be surprised to see how delighted some people are to hear a kind voice while out running their errands or doing their customer service jobs. You may run into a rare cranky person, but don't let them deter you from your mission. Spread some sunshine and feel the glow of that personal interaction as it becomes a natural reflex. Soon, silence will feel uncomfortable as you long for the next chance to chat.

Here are some tips to help you:

- Ask open-ended questions that don't end in a yes or no answer. For example, while it's tempting to keep things short, asking "How are you today?" won't take you far. Instead, start with an observation and invite them to fill in some details, such as "I've noticed you are wearing your hair shorter these days. It looks good on you. Are you trying a new look, or do you want to stay cooler this summer?" Complimenting someone's clothes, pet, or car is also an excellent way to start the ball rolling.

- Relax. If you're tense and clam up after the first exchange, the other person will sense it. Make sure you continue breathing (it's easy to find yourself holding it in) and deliberately unclench your shoulders and hands. These actions send subtle signals to your brain that everything is fine, taking your nervousness down a notch.

- Don't rush to fill the silence. People get restless if they don't get a response right away, but you have to give others a chance to formulate their thoughts. They may have been thinking about something else, listening to music via earbuds you didn't see, or just not be used to strangers chatting them up. It will be worth the wait.

- Smile and remain relaxed and open to listening when they are ready to speak. If all goes well, you may be talking regularly, so tuck what they say into your memory bank for future encounters. When I first moved into my new condo, I would come home, pull out my contact sheet, and write down a name or suite number right away until I knew people and their pets better.

- Focus on the person in front of you. Don't fidget with your bags or your phone. Instead, give them your undivided attention so the other person feels engaged and appreciated.

- Be optimistic. If you expect things to go well, it's more likely they will. By putting out positive vibes, the other person will respond to the energy that you are sharing.

Over time, you will build your confidence, and you will look forward to kibitzing with your neighbors and others who cross your path while you're out and about. You never know when you'll meet a future friend of any gender so stay open to new connections.

GET OUT MORE

Now that you're greeting more people while doing your mundane daily tasks, why not expand your universe to encompass more people? Start calling your friends to get out for coffee and to see how they are doing. Make time for lunch with your siblings or that neighbor you've discovered shares some of your interests. This is another step forward, as you don't wait for others to invite you: you reach out and initiate simple, small gatherings to try out a new restaurant or walk on a trail near your home.

Once this is part of your routine, ask your friends about classes or activities that enrich their lives. You've heard the fuss about yoga but haven't tried it yet; you'd like to see why it is becoming a beloved part of so many people's fitness regimens. You now have the time for golf and welcome a chance to get back into it or another activity like cycling, hiking, or that new Zumba dance class.

Start scoping out what activities are available in your area that you haven't tried yet. If you're short on ideas, here are some resources to get your brain in the right gear:

- Be a tourist in your own town. Go to the tourism office or check its website to see what attractions draw people from other areas. You may have heard about a new outdoor play gym for adults when it opened but never headed there to try it out. Now is your chance.

- Check the listings with your local seniors' center. These facilities are set up for anyone over fifty, so don't think you have to be ancient to enjoy their fitness classes, discussion groups, games, and crafts. They are constantly switching up their offerings to stay current and are open to ideas if you have something in mind. You can dance, play cards, compete at shuffleboard, or even get grief counseling if you shop around.

- Try a new restaurant a couple of times a month. If you're on a budget, treat yourself to breakfast or lunch to keep the cost down, but allow yourself to splurge when you can. You will discover new dishes and flavors while chatting with different servers and clientele during your meals.

- If your town or city has one, check volunteer centers to seek out ways to help out. You can get weekly shifts at certain schools or charities or just sign up for special events. Healthcare services often need volunteer drivers or people to greet people at events. Find a task that meshes with your skills and comfort level; then you'll have a new portal for meeting people.

- If you have mobility issues or you are just not ready to get out in person, try signing up for an online interactive learning platform. For example, GetSetUp is a platform and community specifically designed to help older adults enjoy learning new things and meeting new friends. GetSetUp is making a difference in older adults' lives by socially connecting them through learning and combating social isolation and loneliness. Check them out at www.getsetup.io.

Inch by inch, you will feel your self-esteem grow as you become a bigger part of the world around you. You have so much to offer, so why would you hold it back? There are so many people who have yet to reach your point; by talking with them and making them feel valued and connected, you brighten their days and give them a sense that someone cares about how they feel and look. In return, you get a boost that makes you smile and opens your heart to even more interactions as you reach even further towards your goal.

* * *

WEEK 6 ASSIGNMENTS

❖ Carry on with the tasks from Weeks 1 to 5. Keep flattering yourself by writing good points in your journal, exercising regularly, and clearing out old baggage.

❖ Add more inspirational quotes and affirmations as they come to you, and enjoy each one.

❖ Keep your list of wants, needs, and deal-breakers handy as you watch other couples – real or fictional – to determine what resonates with you.

❖ Every day, find a chance to chat with someone in your circle. If you don't see people in person, dial up an old friend to see how they are.

❖ Set up one to two events this week, such as meeting a friend (new or old) or relative for coffee, a walk, or a casual meal. As one event ends, plan where you want to go next to keep up the momentum. Start stockpiling ideas since you will be continuing this trend from now until the end of the program.

KEY TAKEAWAYS

Practicing your skills at making small talk will make it easier to break the ice with new people, especially if you start small.

You need to get out of your usual spaces to meet new people and open yourself up to new experiences. Go gently, and it will feel more natural as you grow more confident.

* * *

I thought I would take this moment to check in with you. How are you doing? How are you feeling? Has the material and assignments so far given you some direction, hope, and optimism? I truly hope so. Not long ago, I was likely where you are right now.

As a Health & Life Coach, it is important not to leave anyone out. Everyone deserves to live a vibrant life. If this book has opened your mind, brought you some joy, a glimmer of hope, or a solid plan to have more in your life, I have a favor to ask you. Please stop what you are doing right now, and go to your computer or phone and leave a review at your preferred retailer.

Your review will greatly help other readers decide if this book could help them too. Thank you for taking the time to leave a review.

8

HOW TO DATE SMARTLY
(ESPECIALLY ONLINE)

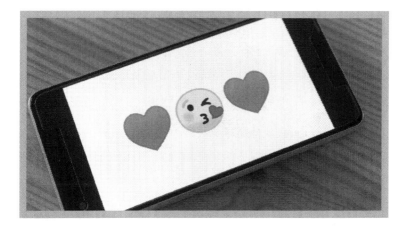

$\mathcal{M}$uch of the buzz about seeking a partner these days focuses on the many online choices, from dedicated dating sites, to sidelines for platforms such as Facebook. While these forums have led to some wonderful outcomes for many couples, it is not the only option out there. I must confess that I met my husband via a dating site, and we are extremely happy together. We are definitely one of the success stories for these companies. I have also met countless couples who wouldn't have found each other without the internet. Your luck is primarily based on who is out there at the same time you are and how you present yourself. One of my friends describes the pool of prospective partners as "shallow and wide." If you cast your net into this sea, it is hard to predict what you will catch.

Of course, if you are averse to using computers, this isn't for you. You can read this chapter for interest's sake or simply skip it. However, it does give you an overview that may be helpful when speaking to friends or family members if they decide to jump onto Plenty of Fish, Match, Christian Mingle, or eHarmony (or the many other websites and apps out there). It may also give you some ideas on presenting yourself in person and what red flags can occur, even when you are dating offline.

Most general dating sites offer a same-sex section where you can look around. If you prefer a same-sex-only site, men can try Adam4Adam, MenNation, or FabGuys, but expect to find a high proportion of younger men there. For women, HER is a site for you. Regardless of what gender you are seeking, the advice of this chapter applies.

THE TOP TEN MISTAKES ONLINE DATERS MAKE

These are not intended to spook you and provide you excuses to give up on your mission. Rather, I would prefer that you have a great experience like I ultimately did when my husband and I crossed paths. Furthermore, by making wise choices at the outset, you are less likely to throw in the towel and miss out on connecting with some people who are compatible with your interests and goals in life.

Don't do these things:

1. Post a photo that says too much

In the digital space, a photo is worth far more than a thousand words. It can be the make-it-or-break-it piece of the puzzle as most people make assessments within a fraction of a second – usually five milliseconds – and decide whether to read about you or to move on. Therefore, you have to make a good first impression with the photo you choose to post as part of your profile. It is incredible what people will post when they are in a rush or don't see the elements of the image that may not represent them well. Learn from their errors:

- Too much information. Even showing too much skin can be a turnoff. Keep your shirt on, and don't flash too much cleavage. It's not a classy move and may turn off someone who is looking for a person for conversation, not just a physical relationship. It also makes you look superficial and overshadows your strengths. Similarly, posting a photo of you in front of your bathroom mirror doesn't reflect that you've put a lot of thought or care into your image. Also, skip any inappropriate clothing. This means no skimpy tank tops or dirty sweatpants since they don't bode well for future decisions. The same goes for the messy bed or couch behind you. Let someone give you a chance before they find out you didn't fold laundry for a few days.

- Leave clues about your past. Crop photos to leave out your ex's hand on your shoulder or parts of other people. It just leads to questions and also looks lazy. Surely you have other photos to post.

- Cover your face with a hat and sunglasses. People want to see your eyes to assess who you are. They may also wonder if you're hiding a bald head. Even if you have a scar or something that makes you insecure, you can present your entire face in a flattering way.

- A blurry image. Either you're not committed enough to take a second shot, or you're trying to erase your wrinkles. Sharpen up and try again.

- A group shot that leaves people guessing which one is you. There is already enough mystery in online dating. If you ask people to figure out which one is you, they will just move on without engaging.

- A moody photo. For heaven's sake, just smile. If you're self-conscious about your teeth, then find another expression that is still welcoming. This isn't really the forum for artistic expression, so don't waste your chance to impress others with how happy you can be.

2. Misspell words in your profile

People judge quickly and even more so online. If you make careless grammatical errors, you may miss out on garnering the attention of say, a retired teacher who loves everything you do, but who also admires strong language skills. This is often a case of rushing or being nervous as you post.

Run your sample through a spelling and grammar check program before sharing it. Always read over your posts and replies to messages a couple of times to ensure you didn't omit a word or use a similar-sounding one. No one expects perfection every time, but make an effort with your grammar. If you don't care about how spelling errors look, some may think, then where else do you slack off in life?

3. Share TOO-personal details

You've just 'met' someone, and you're trashing your ex or telling them too much about your bowel disorder. I'm not sure which one is a bigger turnoff. This type of information sends subtle cues about how your relationship would roll out. Will you complain all the time? Will you be disrespectful if this relationship doesn't pan out? Are you looking for someone to be your nurse?

Likewise, putting personal information about where you live, lunch, or work out gives a spurned online suitor a chance to seek you out beyond the safety of the dating platform. Never provide hints about where they can find you, or you could get caught in a scam or a situation that makes you uncomfortable.

Going back to photos, there is never a good time to exchange nude or semi-nude images. This information could be shared far beyond the two of you and could be used to embarrass or blackmail you. Don't give people ammunition to use against you.

4. Write a profile that sounds like everyone else

As a cynical friend told me after viewing dozens of profiles one day, everyone in the dating world likes to walk on the beach, stay fit, listen to music, and snuggle. Unfortunately, this list is so generic that it tells you nothing, except that the person thinks these clichés work.

You want to stand out as unique. Go back to your cocktail party ice-breaker and think about your reply to "What do you do?" Sparkle right from the outset.

Be a storyteller. Drop in the name of your favorite song or flavor of ice cream since details matter. People scan for information so quickly, so make sure to grab them with your heading.

If you need help to objectively see your unique highlights, ask a trusted friend or relative to help you. Or think about the ideal profile you'd like to read and use that as your guide.

5. Put all your eggs in one basket

You pour your heart and soul into sending a message to someone on the site and get nothing back. You begin to wonder what is wrong with you. Why is no one replying? Relax. The right person for you may be taking a break for a holiday or dealing with a family issue. Sometimes, it takes time to cross paths with your match. Don't rely on one person to make or break your experience. Send out more messages and see what comes back.

6. Lie

Posting a photo from twenty years ago or saying you have a hobby involving activities you may plan to do one day may draw more interest. But what do you do when you say you love to kayak and you get invited out on some white-water? Getting caught is never fun, and it will leave a bad taste for those who find out you have exaggerated or fabricated information. So just say how tall you are, what you like to do, and let the chips fall where they may.

7. Come on too strong

You want people to get to know you before you start sharing information that may turn them off. Context is key to having them see the full portrait of your interests and assets. For example, these may be deal-breakers if someone only sees them in isolation:

- Your strong political views are more likely to turn people off than see you find someone who concurs one hundred percent.

- You are determined to get married within a year, but that may be too fast for others. Meet, see where things go, then set a timeline together. Be honest generally about what you're seeking in terms of a partnership, but don't box people in.

- If you're critical of your ex, why would someone else want to join your pity party? Save some baggage for future trips. Just say your previous relationship had some challenges and you want a fresh start.

- Sarcasm works best in person, not meet-and-greet sites. Your sense of humor may not translate in this forum, so save the sarcasm for later.

8. Sit back and wait

You may be a wallflower in real life, but you will wilt if you take that role in online dating. You may be used to the other person reaching out or setting the pace based on traditional gender roles. However, the rules and roles are different here in that the playing field is more level. Reach out and send messages to people who strike you as interesting. Get on more than one site to improve your odds of finding a compatible partner.

Once you connect, answer messages within a few days and don't keep people guessing by ghosting them. This is not high school where you still see each other in the halls and can play mind games. The other person may just move on after reading your signals as a lack of interest.

Just as we talked about, when it comes to ice-breakers, plant seeds to grow the conversation so the other person doesn't have to do all the work. I know it's hard if you're shy or new to this type of communication. Just write in your voice and be sincere.

9. Be overly critical

You may flip through profile after profile and find fault with all of them. Unfortunately, that just gets you back to square one. Don't dismiss people too quickly. If you see a typo, accept that they might have just made a mistake. Instead, invest the time to read to the end of each profile to get a bigger picture view. Your compatibility may not show up until the last line when they talk about their loyal pet.

You may be tempted to assess someone on looks only. Instead, ask yourself, "Would I want them to do the same?" Go back to your core values and your understanding of what you want and need. After all, love is more than skin deep.

10. Wait too long to act or give up too soon

I almost gave up on my husband-to-be when we continued our online chat for quite some time without him offering to meet for coffee. Now, I know better and could have asked him for coffee myself. Luckily, he invited me out just as I was about to give up hope, and look at how it turned out. I am so happy to have an amazing partner in my life. Having learned from that experience, I would suggest that you set up a meeting after a few exchanges to see if the chemistry online is real or not. Start small with coffee or a walk. If they don't ask you, you can ask them.

If you don't get much interest, keep going. Adapt your profile and add a new photo. Ask a friend to look at your profile to see if something is missing. Your special someone may be on another platform, so try spreading your wings a little further.

On the other end of the spectrum, don't expect each conversation to lead to a marriage proposal. It's a *dating* site. It's helpful to be realistic and not think that you'll find your prince or princess within a week. Be patient.

Now, it may sound like I've taken a negative tone here, but that doesn't mean you cannot have some great experiences with online dating. There are some warm and wonderful people out there who are also trying to connect with reasonable adults with common interests. Unfortunately, there are also a small minority of people looking to take advantage of you, so be aware of these predators before they break your heart and your bank account.

BEWARE OF ROMANCE SCAMMERS

These individuals create fake identities or concoct information about themselves as they flood you with compliments, then ask for money. This is a high-stakes game that, frighteningly, works. In the United States alone, $304 million was taken from love-struck people in 2020, a fifty-percent increase over the previous year.[9] These individuals tend to target older people since they assume that you have accumulated more wealth at this point in your life than someone younger.

These scammers build a bridge first, acting like a normal suitor, but the relationship grows fast.

They are often residents of Third World countries who want to emigrate or individuals who claim to be lonely as they are posted in a job overseas, often with military or medical organizations. They can be very charming and know how to disarm their targets by giving them the responses they think will keep their hooks planted.

There are some commons tactics that may give you a sense if this person is real or posing as a prospective partner:

- They disappear on weekends and make excuses for their absence.

- Their English is written in awkward ways, using expressions that don't sound right. Often, these scammers are working in their second or third language and it shows.

- The first message is generic, as if copied over and over again. For example, "I saw your profile and want to learn more about you." Normally, a person would highlight something you've said or a common interest in hopes of making a connection.

- The photo on their profile changes regularly. Usually, they have copied a photo from a real person's site and may have been caught by another person. If you're suspicious, copy and paste their image into an online search engine to see where else it pops up. This tip is very useful, since you can solve a mystery within a few minutes.

- They try to move your conversation off the dating platform so they can ask you for more personal information without getting caught. Don't get drawn away.

- They profess love sooner than expected. While this is flattering, it is also likely insincere.

- They offer to come to see you but keep canceling. After all, they don't want to end this too quickly.

- They say they need money for a plane ticket, medical expenses, or to clear up a gambling debt. No one should be asking you for money before meeting in person. They may cite the cost of a visa or other documents to travel to see you and say they cannot wait to save up the money. Even if the person is real, do you want to end up with someone who cannot manage their funds well? It could end up as an expensive trap either way.

- They ask you for bank information, passwords, or another secret. Don't give anyone any leverage, especially when it comes to financial information. They can use it to infiltrate your account or blackmail you. Never send nude or semi-nude photos for the same reason. That's just not acceptable for any age.

- They ask for gift cards. These are commodities that can be either bartered or sold for cash. Never give anything valuable to a person you have never met face to face.

If you get caught in this type of web of lies, you may feel embarrassed and want to keep it to yourself. This means that the jerk who did this to you is more likely to get away with it again. Take a deep breath and report the information, along with all your exchanges, to legal authorities, in the interests of protecting others. Also, if you gave money via gift cards, the U.S. Federal Trade Commission advises you to contact the company that was the unsuspecting intermediary and ask them to void the transaction so you can get your money back.

If you feel uncomfortable with a person on a dating website, stop communicating with them. Instead, trust your instincts and keep on fishing. This point is so important. Listen to your gut.

Now that you have a good grasp of what conversations you're having online, let's move on to some key communication you'll have in person – broaching the subject of dating with your friends and family.

GO PUBLIC

You don't want your adult children to find out you're dating from someone else, like an in-law who sees your profile pop up in their feed. Wouldn't that be awkward? Now that you're about to start reaching out to other people, you may want to inform your family and close friends that you've decided to fill this void in your life and that you would like their support. You may be surprised at how helpful they will be.

It may take some of them some time to get used to the idea, so let them percolate. You don't need to change course if you meet some reticence. Listen to what they have to say and respond accordingly. They may be used to you living on your own and being available to help them at all times. Or they may worry about you losing your financial independence. Appreciate their concern and reassure them as needed.

This may open up the door for people around you to introduce you to friends that may be suitable suitors for you. You have now expanded your search to yet another platform. You could also double-date with friends if you're nervous about going out one on one. Look at all the pluses and benefit from them. You may also enlist friends and family to help you take a flattering photo or offer their technical skills to show you how to create shortcuts to your Match profile. Make them part of the mission.

By now, I hope you are feeling braver, confident, stronger, and wiser as you firm up exactly what you are looking for in a mate and where to go looking. With your life free of emotional and physical clutter, you have your sights set forward.

* * *

WEEK 7 ASSIGNMENTS

❖ Carry on with the tasks from Weeks 1 to 6. Keep writing in your journal, getting out to exercise, and seeking out positive affirmations.

❖ Keep reading, being grateful, and seeking ways to get out of the house to spread joy to people around you.

❖ Commit to joining one regular activity outside of the house. You've already gone out for lunch, but now you need a club or a course to learn something new and connect with people in a shared setting. There are endless possibilities, so keep an open mind.

KEY TAKEAWAYS

Online dating has connected countless couples and is a place where you can safely meet nice people.

Avoiding common mistakes in online dating will make it a more rewarding and fruitful experience for you.

Romance scams do happen, but there are clear signs that are easy to identify once you know what they are.

9

SEEK YOUR TARGET-RICH
ENVIRONMENT (OFFLINE)

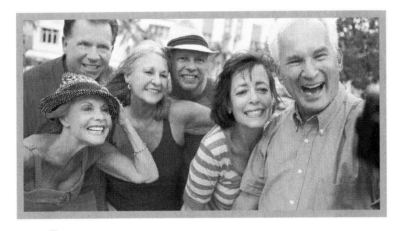

*Y*ears ago, I heard the term 'target-rich environment' while watching an interview with Dr. Phil, the TV relationship guru, who outlined the idea in his 2005 book *Love Smart: Find the One You Want; Fix the One You've Got*. To illustrate his point, on his TV show, he took a pair of women named Stacey and Jo-Anne to places where they were likely to find men: a bookstore and the batting cages.[10] He reasoned that it made more sense to go where the men were in order to improve your odds of meeting one. After all, he said, it's not like the right person is going to walk up to your front steps and randomly knock on your door while you languish inside in your sweatpants.

It was pretty pragmatic advice that seemed to work for Stacey as she made eye contact with a man who was interested in her. For the second step, Dr. Phil made sure the women were equipped with opening lines to deepen the interest of the men they met.[11] Again, it seems obvious, but who actually does that?

You do. Starting today.

Think about where you and your friends met your previous partners. You were likely in school together, at a party full of people, or working with individuals who were close in age and proximity. You were surrounded by prospects, and you talked with a bunch of them before you homed in on whichever person you liked the most. Things progressed from there. Now you need to repeat that process.

It is unlikely that you are going to find a college class full of sixty-year-olds, so that location goes off the list. Yet, you will find yourself among your peers if you take an exercise class in the middle of the day, or head to the community center for midday dancing, or take up a hobby-related club that someone your age invited you to join. Even if there are younger people in that setting, they may have a relative who would be a nice match for you. Remember, you are spreading the word that you are available and on the market, so keep talking yourself up, no matter where you go.

If you choose to stay home and clean out your closets, you are shutting yourself off from the outside world. How can you possibly meet Mr. or Mrs. Right if you are playing hide and seek without them even knowing you exist? I'm exaggerating to reinforce the point. Get out of the house and go where you'll find people like you. It's really that simple.

Go back and look at your list of joyous moments. That should inspire you to decide where you will go on your quest. If travel was high among your priorities, then book a trip with a group or to a location that is popular with your peers. This could vary, depending on how active you are, so I'm not going to set any parameters.

If you're still taking long cycling holidays, then hit the open road with other riders. If you are too arthritic for active travel, book a bus trip where you can sit in comfort while you chat with your seatmates. Make sure you work your way around the group to meet everyone.

Closer to home, brainstorm where else you expect to find people with similar interests and lifestyles. I'll get you started, but feel free to add to my ideas:

- A coffee shop with other morning people
- A library or bookstore for other avid readers
- The gym for active athletes
- Community dances where you can attend with a group of friends
- Clubs, for crafts or collecting
- Film festivals for cinephiles
- Tai chi and yoga classes
- Horticulture clubs for those with green thumbs
- The golf course during the day
- Theaters (as a patron or behind the scenes as a volunteer)
- A continuing-education class on memoir-writing or other skills
- At the hospital as a volunteer
- A church, synagogue, or mosque, either at services or during committee work

Of course, you continue asking friends to keep you in mind in case they run into an old friend who is also single. Networking is key to getting more people to know you so they can recommend you as a pleasant person to spend time with.

FUN AND DIFFERENT DATE IDEAS

Once you meet someone, you'll want to find unique ways to spend your time together, so you don't end up in a rut. After all the work you've done to expand your horizons, you want to make the most of your mindset and explore even further. You can start with simple pleasures, like a coffee, walk, or lunch. However, it can get stale quickly if you get set in your ways without having a little fun first.

Since you have committed to being physically active, you can kill two birds with one stone if you get in a golf game or a yoga class together. Activities done together also build up a strong camaraderie, especially if there is physical contact. Get your heart pumping and those endorphins may help you connect more deeply with the person you're with.

Here are some ideas to keep moving and having fun. Even if you haven't found your special someone yet, you can always keep these options open for when you do:

- Pull out those lawn games you used to love and play like a kid again. Croquet calls on a series of skills, and you can rib each other as you each take the lead. A game of horseshoes is also fun but needs a specific setup. Bocce is low maintenance if you have access to a set of balls and a level lawn.

- Go dancing. Even if you're not Ginger Rogers and Fred Astaire, you'll still enjoy the music. Once you get talking about your favorite tunes, you may not even get up and boogie. However, the option is always there.

- Ride your bikes. Pick a trail and go out and explore. With the advent of e-bikes, it's easier than ever to go out and pedal while having a backup system if you push yourself too far. Plan out stops along the way to rest and refuel.

- Shoot pool. Billiards is a challenge for your mind and your balance as you figure out how to work the angles around the table. Again, you can have a little competition without raising the stakes too high.

- Tour a brewery or a winery. This is really just an excuse for a road trip, but it's a good one. These facilities are often based on rural properties where you can also hike and explore where the grapes or hops are grown. You'll get exposed to new sights and tastes that will fill your senses.

- Pick berries. Eating food that you harvested makes you appreciate it even more. Grab some baskets and fill them up with tasty treats. If bending over is a problem, wait until autumn when most apple crops are ready. You can simply pull them from the trees and enjoy their sweetness with your sweetheart.

- Do a photoshoot. Pick a scenic location and look at it at various angles with your cameras in hand. You will each see things the other misses, so you can guide each other along the way. Of course, you can also take pictures of each other to treasure.

As you can see, you are limited only by your imagination. I hope this also reminds you how much fun it is to share your days with another adventurer.

WEEK 8 ASSIGNMENTS

❖ Carry on with the tasks from Weeks 1 to 7. Stay positive and active as you embrace new places and opportunities.

❖ Find new books to read and new faces to pepper with compliments. Your mind and your circle of influence should be growing.

❖ Keep finding reasons to leave the house and meet new people. Identify target-rich environments and go there regularly to interact with people. Don't be too shy or you'll defeat your purpose of going out in the first place.

❖ Get a current photo of yourself while out doing activities you enjoy. You can hire a professional, take a selfie, or ask a friend or relative to help you. Choose a setting that makes you smile, preferably in natural light that flatters you.

KEY TAKEAWAYS

You can only meet people in real life if you leave your home and your comfort zone to encounter them.

By going to a target-rich environment, you increase your odds of meeting people who share your interests.

Identify places you can go and things you can do to enrich your life, both while you search for a partner and when you actually find someone.

10

SEEK YOUR TARGET-RICH ENVIRONMENT (ONLINE)

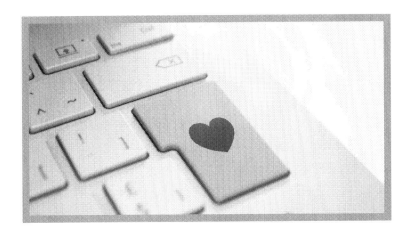

*O*kay, you're feeling energized and full of ideas of the fun things that will brighten up your life. Your home is uncluttered and you've swept away any emotional baggage to make room for new experiences. Now, let's see who is out there beyond your usual social networks.

If you are nervous about online dating, take a deep breath and ask yourself what is making you hesitate. Years ago, everyone was hesitant to shop online or do their banking from home, but now it is an everyday habit. Dating sites thrive because there is a need for people to meet and because they have made it as welcoming and successful as they can.

As a veteran of this experience, I will walk you through it so you know where to go and what to do. The mistakes from Chapter 8 were presented so you know what not to do. Now let's talk about what to do and how. Before we get there, here's a little romance to inspire you.

Peter was a retired college professor in a small city where he hadn't met anyone with his flair for international travel and cuisine. He was born in Europe and often returned there for work, so he wasn't inspired by cruises or trips to Caribbean resorts. Once he expanded his search via an online dating platform, he met Lillian, who lived about a hundred miles away. Soon, they were shopping at markets and batch cooking together. Once she retired as well, she moved to his home and they are living happily ever after.

Meanwhile, Emily had pretty much given up on guys after repeatedly reuniting and splitting with her long-time partner. She was having a hard time getting him out of her mind. She tried online dating and met a few incompatible matches over the first year. She was about to give up when a quirky smile caught her eye. When she read Tom's profile, she found out he was a juggler and she couldn't resist sending him a message.

Two years later, they still see each other on weekends and talk during the week as they live separate lives. However, she and Tom are both ecstatic to have someone to call when they've had a tough day or a great experience. He is even teaching her how to juggle!

And finally, Andrew had had a crush on Tony for years, but they hadn't seen each other since they were both dating mutual friends. Andrew's heart nearly jumped out of his chest when he saw a familiar face on his computer screen when he was surfing for dates online. The two connected and were married last year. It turns out Tony had wanted to ask Andrew out years before, but didn't think he was interested. It was a pleasant surprise for both men to find out how quickly they clicked and created a cozy home together.

WHERE DO YOU START?

The first step toward finding your mate – in whatever form you've decided works for you – is to determine what you're going to say in your introduction. This is a virtual cocktail party, so don't try to blend in with the crowd. This is your chance to share what makes you so unique. If you make the best butter tarts in the world, sweeten your profile with that information. If you love to dance to a specific type of music, play up your moves. Even if you are a quiet bookworm, you can talk about the stories that keep you up all night, tearing through the pages.

If you are struggling to get the right words down, remember everyone has a hard time selling themselves.

Ask your fans to help you. Turn to a trusted friend or a supportive sister-in-law to help you see what you are too close to see for yourself. They may boost your confidence by telling you how they have always admired your smile or point out an attribute that you have taken for granted. Voilà, you now have something to highlight. (Of course, you can add in juggling, since it worked out so well for Tom.)

Next, you want to craft a narrative that will draw the right type of attention. You begin with the heading that says just as much with its tone as it does with the facts within it. For inspiration, here are some original ones:

- Music Lover Looking to Write the Next Verse
- Art-Loving Women: Let's Paint a Picture of Life Together
- Casting Call for Movie Buffs! Send Me Your Favorite Movie Quote
- Math Nerd Looking for Someone to Add to My Life and Multiply the Fun
- Tired of Online Dating? Let's Be Each Other's Reason for Signing Off[12]

Don't those give you a sense of the person's interests and their sense of humor? That is the kind of wording that makes people smile, which is the key to making a connection. If you are stuck, go back to your lists of positive traits or inspiring quotes to see which words resonate when you think about the initial signal you wish to send. Brainstorm a few and ask a friend if you're torn between options and need a nudge to pick one out. However, don't feel so pressured that you have to earn a Pulitzer Prize the first time out. You may refine your heading as you learn the dynamics of each site and find that certain words work better as time goes on.

The next part should be easier, since you've already decided which part of wonderful you will be highlighted. From here, it could be easy to fall into the trap of describing your traditional roles within your family or career, but resist that urge. Instead, focus on your passions and let that energy shine through.

Imagine you are writing a biography that will appear on a book jacket or at the start of a course. You can mention professional details, but that spark is what people really want to see to discover what is below the surface. Skip the urge to include every fact about yourself. This isn't a list of your skills and talents; it's a snapshot of your personality. Look at other profiles to see what others are saying. I'll give you the menu of the best sites for people over sixty in a moment.

Also, be proud of who you are. Put it out there that you just nailed that new yoga pose, or you've read every James Patterson novel ever published. Make sure every word is sincere and avoid clichés: people will see right through them, and it doesn't tell them what they need to know. Make it glow with positivity and add specific details about flavors, hobbies, and favorite things. Proofread it and run it through a grammar check to make sure it reads well. Flip back a couple of chapters to see the list of mistakes and learn from them. Limit your personal information and focus on your unique qualities.

Don't put your deal-breakers out there quite yet, since you want to focus on what you want, not what turns you off. There is no need to be modest. Make them fall in love with you.

Now, pick the photos you want to share, leading with your strongest one. They should show a smiling, in-focus, and active you, living your life with gusto. Wear a bright color to grab their attention and crop the image, so your face is the most prominent part.

WHERE DO I PUT IT?

Of all the dating sites out there, I would recommend these five, since they have a robust community of people who use them, and the sites are very credible. They have been doing this for a long time and they know just how to adjust algorithms to put the right people together. Start with one site to get comfortable, then try others as you get used to checking messages and increase your comfort level. Only you know which one is best suited for you.

Match – If you love to shop around to see who is out there, this long-time veteran of the dating game is a good start. After twenty years of making matches, it has several thousand profiles and will present you within the feeds of people looking for love. It is more open-ended than other sites that dial you into people who share your specific interests. You can use the free version, but it's not as effective as the paid version. If you don't meet someone special in the first six months, your next six months are free.

eHarmony – This is probably the smartest site since it goes deep right from the outset and narrows the field right away. You do an extensive personality test to hone in on how you communicate, your key characteristics, what drives you, and how you organize your daily life. If that doesn't define you, then I'm not sure what would. Again, you can go with a free option, but the paid one is more efficient at finding people willing to spend a few bucks just to meet you. If money is tight, ask about its reduced monthly rate.

Silver Singles – This site also runs you through an in-depth questionnaire when you sign up, to focus on your personality and how you live your life. It feeds you five matches per day, which is a good pace for a beginner. With mature members only, you will only meet people in your age range.

Senior Match – If you're looking for a friend for travel or other activities your friends don't enjoy, this is the place for those casual relationships. You may still find more, if that's what you're seeking. Everyone here is over the age of forty-five, so that weeds out people who may be too young for you, depending on your parameters.

Our Time – For a relaxed atmosphere, you can peruse the profiles of people looking for love or look out for someone seeking a sidekick for travel. This is only for people over fifty and tends to draw more active people.

You can also try Plenty of Fish or Zoosk to spread your net even further.

Like every person profiled, these sites each have their own personality. You can also get recommendations from friends who are shopping around too. Once you get used to the sites, just like Facebook, you'll be using them regularly to keep tabs on your contacts in a friendly way.

KEEP IT FRESH

As you 'meet' and talk with your matches, stay attuned to which parts of your profile they mention in their responses and which ones they don't. That is a guide for tweaking your profile to add new information you think would be of interest. It's often the specifics that speak to people who like the same things that you do.

Carry your camera with you so you don't have any regrets when you find yourself in a setting that lights up your smile. Ask friends to keep taking photos that you can add to your profile. The best photos arise from times when you are relaxed and enjoying yourself, whether it's after a hike or a latte on a patio. Current images are also more honest than that stunning portrait from when you were twenty years younger and a few pounds lighter. This is who you are. Anyone would be lucky to befriend you.

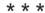

WEEK 9 ASSIGNMENTS

❖ Carry on with the tasks from Weeks 1 to 8. Keep focusing on staying active, in terms of exercise, socializing with friends, and weekly activities.

❖ Read new books and watch out for more inspirational posts to keep you energized. By now, these habits should be part of your routine as you continue to learn about yourself and the world around you.

❖ Keep seeking out target-rich places to shop and spend your social time. Try new stores, even if you're just browsing. Ask your friends where they see people like the mates you are seeking and follow their advice. By now, people should know you're up for dating, so make them your allies (and your scouts!)

❖ Create your online dating profile without overthinking it. Have fun with your drafts and pick out the photos that you feel portray the inner you. You can tweak it after the first draft, but take that first step to figure out which platforms work for you and how they work. Again, you will learn as you go.

KEY TAKEAWAYS

If you feel hesitant to post an online profile, ask yourself what is holding you back. Look at the positives and give it a try.

Get help from people who admire you if you find it hard to 'sell' yourself. You have many great qualities; you just have to pick which ones to highlight.

The different types of sites can restrict or open up your options, depending on which one(s) you choose. Start with one and expand when you're ready.

You can always update and improve your profile: see what resonates with the people you talk to and add to those elements. Keep taking new photos to share and smile. You're really doing this. What an awesome achievement!

11

DON'T GET OBSESSED

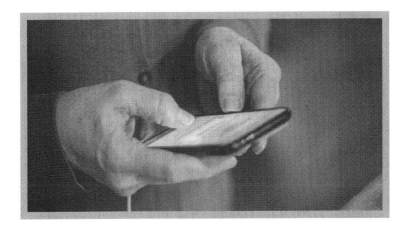

As soon as Vicky saw Daniel's profile, she felt an instant connection. His looks and his smile seemed to beam right through her fog of doubt about online dating. She messaged him right away. In fact, the words seemed to fly out of her fingers as she talked about their common interests. When he replied with interest, she was over the moon.

Soon, she was dreaming about their life together and planning when she could travel to meet him. She kept these thoughts to herself as she tried to gauge how interested he was in her. The time between messages seemed like an eternity. To pass the time, she read them over and over again, then started searching for him on social media. She asked him more probing questions about his life in hopes of ferreting out more clues about his personal information.

When he went quiet and left the platform, she felt the loss deeply and was disoriented. What had she done wrong? Could she have reacted differently? Her confidence plummeted and she ignored messages from other possible suitors. On a rational level, Daniel may have found love with someone else, but Vicky couldn't see that side quite yet. She felt she had failed, and it took her more than a month before she rebounded and tried again. This time, she was more careful about investing her emotions right away. While it took her another month before she found a spark with another man, it was worth the wait. They are faithful companions to each other, even while living apart across an international border.

Whether you're meeting people online or in person, moderation is key. If you overdo it, you may lose your perspective and undermine some of the groundwork you've done to get to this point. In other words, there is no need to get obsessed.

If you dedicate your life to this mission, you will get demoralized. Don't check your inbox every five minutes. Getting too into the 'game' can prevent you from seeing red flags, or even the yellow ones.

It's easy to get caught up in seeing how many profiles you can check or messages you will receive. However, quality is more important than quantity. If you like someone who doesn't respond, just let them go rather than stalking their profiles or researching them on other platforms. Focus more on the people who want you to be in their lives.

MAKING DATING A HEALTHY HABIT

Make it a habit to check in with your dating platform for **no more than an hour a day.** Treat it like brushing your teeth. You can clean them up in a couple of minutes, so why scrub away for longer than you need? A one-hour check-in allows you to catch up on messages in a reasonable time frame, but it also gives you time to reflect on who you have seen and how you would like to proceed.

Most people will be willing to wait a day or two to hear from you, and likewise, you would probably prefer a partner who has a full life of their own. Typically, you want to make the switch from typing chat messages to talking face to face within three weeks.

Here are ten other tips to help you make the most of your time online to sift through all the information in front of you carefully yet efficiently:

· · ·

1. Read between the lines

The tone of a person's profile will tell you more about them than the actual words. "I am smart" doesn't resonate if their sentences don't make sense; likewise, you'll find out if they have a sense of humor if a quip resonates. Ultimately, you want to find someone likable and doesn't need to impress you with a long list of degrees or certifications.

Trust your intuition as you seek out someone with character traits – not just hobbies – that match your own. You can even ask, "What did you see in my profile that prompted you to reach out?" That cuts to the chase and tells you if they picked up on your cleavage or your charm. It also tests to see if they read it or just clicked on the message or match icon for everyone in their feed.

2. Give people a chance

There is a profile that keeps floating up, thanks to the algorithm, that is poorly written or has a corny joke in it that makes you roll your eyes. However, there is a reason why it's on your radar. Don't be too quick to dismiss it based on a quick read. Some people stink at writing profiles but could make great partners. However, if your gut says a firm 'no' due to a racist statement or an obvious values mismatch, kiss them goodbye.

This isn't a rom-com where the music will swell up when you meet the right person. Remind yourself that sometimes it takes time to build chemistry. It may take a few awkward conversations until you find your groove. In the meantime, enjoy getting to know each other. Listen to the other person's answers without focusing on how you look in the video box. Ask open-ended questions to give them a chance to really reveal what makes them tick. Then decide how you feel.

3. Don't lower your bar

After a few false starts, you are not finding the type of person you had hoped to encounter. You decide he or she does not exist and change your parameters to open up to more options. Yikes! Now you're being flooded with incompatible people and you have to turn them down. This is no fun either.

After you've done the work to decide who you want in your life, there is no need to change your mind due to a few slow weeks. You are in this for the long run, so remind yourself to be patient and that you deserve the best match possible. Keep that bar high and soon you will find new faces in your feed.

4. Be yourself

When you get nervous during a first-time experience, it's common to talk in a different voice, whether it's faster or higher. You could easily fall into the same trap when you chat online. It's tempting to try to become what you think the other person wants you to be. But how can you meet the right person if you don't act like yourself?

Don't put up a false front. That shows insecurity and may lead to you partnering up with someone who is not respectful of who you are and what you stand for. You don't want others to be fake with you, so resist the urge to fall into a 'role' as a single woman or man in the dating world. Be your wonderful, authentic you to meet your true match.

5. Don't dawdle

If you keep chatting online and don't make the leap to a video or in-person meeting, your matches may lose hope and move on. After a few digital exchanges, set up a short video chat to see if you have a rapport when you hear each other's voices and look into each other's eyes. This is a great precursor to any physical meeting, which is hard to end if you've ordered a meal, bought a movie ticket, or booked a trip to meet them.

This also gives you a chance to find out if your new friend is really who they say they are. Nothing works quicker to cut to the heart of a scam than to ask your potential partner to show their face. Even if the other person is legit, it's harder for them to lie in person about what they've told you. If they have raved about their beloved pet as a selling point, here's where you find out if Rover is real.

People tend to touch their faces when they fib (or may have another 'tell' like a stammer or lack of blinking) so watch for those cues. They may also fidget more or dart their eyes. Use your common sense and ask questions. You can always go back and check your chats if they say something that isn't consistent with a previous conversation.

Take charge and push to take the next step without waiting too long. Hearing the other person's voice and seeing their smile in real time can really open your eyes about how you feel about them.

6. Practice, practice, practice

If this sounds familiar, that's because it repeats the notion that beginning more conversations becomes more natural the more you do it. Your first message exchanges and video chats may feel excruciating – but they do get better with time. Not only will you become more comfortable with the technology, but you will also learn what works and what doesn't.

Perhaps you had an anecdote that you thought would brighten the conversation, but it fell flat. Or perhaps a random comment opened up a whole new insightful discussion. You'll also discover the clues that bring your deal-breakers to the surface; that's worth a few practice calls alone.

Learn as you go and forgive yourself for any early gaffes. If you accidentally hung up on the first call, you can laugh about it later. It does get easier, I promise.

7. Have real conversations

Talking about the weather is only going to get you so far. Once you know how many kids they have and where they worked for most of their careers, it's time to go deeper. You want to find out what you have in common besides the number of birthday cards you buy in a year.

Ask your new acquaintance to describe a perfect day in their own words. What do they want to be famous for? If they could change anything about the way they were raised, what would it be? What do they value most in a friendship? Tell them your life story in four minutes. These examples arise from the "36 questions: How to fall in love" from the *New York Times,* in case you want to read the whole list. This exercise encourages you to take turns asking these types of questions to learn how the other person sees the world.

8. Make sure you're on the same page

If you're looking for a casual travel partner, don't feel pressured into more just to make the other person like you. Just because the first people you meet want a long-distance relationship when you don't, doesn't mean you have to give in. Extricating yourself from someone else's expectations takes a lot of energy and dexterity, so don't put yourself in that awkward position. You should have stated in your profile what you're seeking so anyone who has read it fully will know where you stand.

Typically, men are more likely to ask if your definition of a relationship includes sex. If a man does ask you, be clear with your wishes, whether it's a yes, no, or just not yet. We'll be talking about intimate relationships in the next chapter.

9. End every interaction on a high note

Even if things didn't go as planned, thank the person for their time or mention the highlight of your discussion. Make them feel valued, since they may prove to be worth a second date when you look back later. You know the expression that people may not remember what you said, but they will recall how you made them feel. Hang onto some friendly or positive comments for your wrap-up, since that is what will most likely stick in the other person's mind.

If you accidentally hit the wrong button, send a quick message to rebuild the bridge between you. Then make sure you check back in within a week to see if they want to talk further. Also, remember to set up plans for what comes next, so no one is left hanging. Say, "I'll message you in a few days" or "Why don't we meet here again on Wednesday?" That takes the stress out of guessing if you're going to disappear from view or not.

10. Have fun

When you dated in your younger years, you knew you would have some encounters that didn't lead anywhere but that still generated great memories. Keep those moments in mind as you 'test-drive' each person you meet. Rather than stressing out about picking 'the right one,' revel in meeting new people who also have a zest for life. Tell stories and reminisce about happier times in your life. Share your favorite one-liners from songs or TV shows. Laugh a little.

Use flattery specifically without going over the top. Tell them if a color looks good on them but don't prattle on about how you don't usually get the attention of such an attractive or accomplished person. Even your gossip should be positive and upbeat. Who wants to spend time with a critic or a curmudgeon? A rare soul, that's who.

Show this person your best traits and demonstrate why they would want to invest more minutes in you. Either of you can decide to move on, but at least you'll know you've given it your best shot.

Remember, you have a great life, so continue to enjoy all the great things you have on the go beyond your dating life. Continue to move every day, so you'll be limber when you start getting out even more. Invite friends over for a meal and keep creating new social connections wherever you go. Don't be shy to invite friends that are a couple to your home. You will be dining with a companion yourself soon.

WEEK 10 ASSIGNMENTS

❖ Carry on with the tasks from Weeks 1 to 9. On top of the fun things listed in the previous paragraph, tackle new book titles and keep your energy up with exercise and aspirations.

❖ Keep visiting target-rich places in case you meet an intriguing person there. If you don't, you're still honing your conversation skills that you can use in other settings.

❖ Update your online dating profile based on any points that seem to resonate with people when they message you. Add more fun photos as you build your collection. This will give your fans new material to admire.

❖ Keep track of how much time you spend on your online dating activities. It's surprising how time can slip away. If it's more than an hour a day, dial it back. Taking a balanced approach is better for you in the long run.

KEY TAKEAWAYS

Learning to limit your online dating time is healthier than obsessing over your messages.

Trust your gut when you talk with people to find out if they are honest and reflect the values you're seeking.

Stand up for what you want and pursue it once you feel the urge to meet with someone by video or in person. Stay positive in every interaction, since you are a class act!

12

LEARN FROM YOUR EXPERIENCES

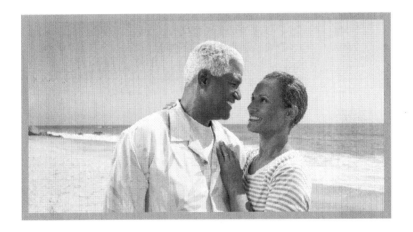

Adam had been on his own for a while and was really enjoying getting out of the house and mingling with the new women he was meeting. It had taken his heart a long time to recover from the loss of the woman he considered the love of his life, but he could feel himself really coming back to life again.

He was laughing and chatting with a few people, drawing on his wit and charm – and realizing how much he had missed sharing this part of himself. He danced. He told jokes and reveled in the laughter of his new friends. He loved having a reason to dress up as he pulled out his favorite suit jackets and golf shirts after they had been hanging sadly in his closet for so long.

Over the next few months, he faced many decisions about how far to go with each of the women he dated, referring back to his list of wants, needs, and deal-breakers. That guided many of his decisions:

- Betty was a great cook and loved to play golf with Adam. However, she was too clingy and wanted him to stop seeing other women and just focus on her right from the outset. He simply wasn't ready to narrow his choices before really getting a chance to meet more people. That was a deal-breaker and they parted ways.

- Ruth loved to eat out at cheap lunch places that mainly served unhealthy choices. As a lifelong athlete, Adam was too health-conscious to order the more popular menu items and soon tired of the same salad over and over again. That ended that partnership. While she 'got' his jokes, she wasn't willing to change her habits to take away the treat of eating out.

- Carol was stunning but she lived in Florida for half of the year, largely for health reasons. Adam didn't want to be apart from a potential partner for that long and didn't choose to travel with her, since it would take him away from his grandchildren.

As hard as it was to step back from these initial matchups, Adam made some tough choices as guided by his principles. He simply wasn't compatible with any single one within this trio, so he kept getting out and connecting with others. For him, dating was more of an exploration than a chore.

He heard fantastic stories about international travel and mischievous grandchildren. He played more golf than he had done in years and had a chance to try out new restaurants. He even made new male friends when he met his dates' brothers or the partners of their long-time female friends. Overall, he was more social, more engaged in the world around him, and enjoying his new life.

He was also learning so much about himself. At this age, Adam was far more aware of how he treated people than when he was younger. All the lessons he had taught his children and grandchildren now returned to him as he practiced patience and kindness with those around him. He rediscovered his love for hobbies he had given up and had now renewed.

INTIMACY WITH A NEW PARTNER

Even as he enjoyed the happy moments, Adam (and probably his partners too) did get stressed about the idea of showing his body and having physical relationships at first. In the beginning, he was self-conscious about his wrinkles, saggy midriff, and surgical scars. Up until this point in his life, only his wife, the guys at the gym, and his doctor had seen him without his clothes on. The idea of undressing in front of another woman for the first time had him breaking out in a cold sweat. He also worried about erectile dysfunction or what would happen if he got sick early on in a new relationship. Would his new partner bail on him? All these questions raced through his mind as he tried to avoid the distraction of his worries.

Let me point out first, though, intimacy is more than just sex. It can be expressed in several ways, including closeness to one another, a deep and meaningful connection, honesty between partners, or simply being in a loving relationship with or without sex. Intimacy, in general, is a great contributor to a sense of belonging and quality of life.

Having intimacy with a partner requires each of you to share parts of yourself with each other. The important factor here is that your sharing is reciprocal and this is why such a bond may become the beautiful, supportive companionship many of us desire. So, please don't let your fear of getting naked in front of a new partner scare you. You will know if, or when, you are ready for this type of intimacy.

Since we have brought it up, let's talk more about sexual intimacy, something Adam worried about.

Generally, most people over the age of sixty who are in relationships report having sex at least once a month.[13] Most of them would like to do it more!

As our bodies change, there are many processes we would like to stop or slow down. Some of them are only skin deep – such as hair loss and tooth extraction – yet others can affect our bond with our partners. Here are some that you may encounter, with tips on how to work around them or at least broach the subject with a new sex partner. It should go without saying that you should talk to your doctor or nurse practitioner about any health issues affecting your quality of life. While you may worry about a partner's reaction, a medical professional has probably heard it all by now and can help you manage or treat the real problem.

Weakened pelvic floor

Dropping hormone levels don't just give us more belly and less physical strength, but they also undermine the structure of the connective tissue in our pelvic area. This happens to three in ten women.[14] That could make it harder to hold your urine, or allow your organs to droop further within your abdomen. In some cases, this may require surgery to prevent interference with your body's normal functions (at a rate of one out of ten women).

You can fight back by drinking eight to ten glasses of water per day and going to the bathroom when you need to. Cutting down other beverages, including coffee and booze, takes away some of the irritants. You can also calm your bladder by eating less fruit and fewer tomato-based dishes. Your other secret weapon is doing exercises like Kegel clenches and pelvic bridges.

If you are beyond that point and rely on incontinence pads, don't give up on a physical relationship out of embarrassment. Wait until you've become comfortable enough with a prospective partner before you have this conversation. This same advice applies to most of the points below.

Back or joint pain

If you struggle to stay upright just to walk around the house, you may find it unimaginable to go through the movements of various intimate positions. By now, you probably have your favorites anyway, but here are the ones that work best to save you from calling for an ambulance mid-coitus:

- The typical man-on-top position can put stress on the woman's back or the man's upper-body joints. To modify it, the woman can lie at the edge of the bed on some pillows while the man stands.

- If the man is less mobile, he can lie on the bottom while the woman is on top and has more control. Since she is kneeling and can lean back or forward on her hands, she has more support.

- For those who are overweight or have hip problems, having the man enter the woman from behind while she is on her hands and knees can be an easier approach. However, it can be hard on your back. It does work for a man in a wheelchair if his partner sits partly in his lap while leaning her arms on the bed to move.

Remember, you can still have a sexual relationship without intercourse. There are many positions where you can engage your hands to stimulate your partner's hot spots, including spooning.

Vaginal dryness

After menopause, women produce less estrogen, making the vaginal walls thinner, less elastic, and drier. It can make sex less stimulating or even painful. This can be disappointing for both partners as it can lower sexual desire and thus frequency. This can be helped by using a water-based lubricant, either from an adult shop or a drugstore.

You can also order a lubricant online if you are shy to buy it in person. Lubricants come in different flavors or with additives that make them feel hot or cool, so have fun while you try them out. Treating it like an experiment will take the pressure off everyone.

Erectile dysfunction

As men age, less blood and testosterone flows to their genitals and they have a harder time achieving and maintaining an erection. This can feel emasculating and disappointing for a couple who hope to have intercourse as part of their relationship.

To keep things flowing, exercise and quit smoking. Carrying less weight and having a healthy heart help to pump blood and hormones when you need them.[15] This means eating a nutritious diet rich in vegetables, lean proteins and whole grains, while rarely drinking.

Memory loss

One of the most frustrating experiences might be the inability to remember details while you are dating someone. At first, it might not be a big deal, but time after time, if one of you is forgetting important things such as a birthdate or where you took your last vacation together, it may start to affect the relationship, including intimacy.

In a more serious circumstance, you may have a partner not remember you. One couple I've met hit a huge rift when a woman, discovered later to have early-onset dementia, started to act strange, sometimes not recognizing her partner. Although this seems like an unlikely scenario, such a situation could occur with dementia appearing on the rise.

My only advice is to enjoy each other's company while you can and talk through how you feel as the situation evolves. The longer you're together, the easier it will be to draw on the memories of the good times to sustain you.

When you begin a relationship, it helps to keep in mind that you may develop a health problem or other medical condition that affects intimacy. Your partner will likely appreciate your empathy based on what you've learned in this chapter.

Just like any other aspect of your relationship, how intimate you become will be part of the negotiation. Don't take it off the table due to worries about not having the physique you did when you started dating decades ago. Unless you're dating someone far younger than you are, it's likely you are both equally uncomfortable or self-conscious.

Your movement and any exercise program should have given you more body awareness, so celebrate your strength. You may not be entering a bathing-suit-model contest, but you are focusing on being more mobile and agile, which can pay off in bed (or on the edge of the bed, as we discussed).

Start small by holding hands, kissing, and sharing secrets as you build trust. Those first steps will help you assess how safe and free you will feel when you're with this person. Without that basis, you may not have a fulfilling physical relationship anyway. Some people can bounce from partner to partner, but you need to know if that works for you at this stage of your life.

WEEK 11 ASSIGNMENTS

❖ Yikes, we only have one left! Carry on with the tasks from Weeks 1 to 10. By now, you should be naturally finding and clearing items you don't need while picking up books and inspirational quotes effortlessly. Keep focusing on removing parts of your unwanted past as you build your brain for an optimistic future.

❖ Get out of the house to enjoy people and activities that infuse you with life, especially areas and interests that may have you crossing paths with a new partner.

❖ Check in on your online dating network daily unless you feel like you need to pause to develop something deeper with one person – either in person or online. Only you will know when to stop shopping, but it doesn't hurt to look around, as long as you're only having dates on a superficial level. Once things get more intense, you'll have to make a decision.

❖ Reassess your wants, needs, and deal-breaker lists as you meet people and discover how much they still fit their respective categories. Maybe your online matches have opened your eyes to how much you had committed to sticking to your guns. Based on your experience, you may wish to tighten the rules or bend them a little more. This is an excellent time to do a reality check, so you can be more pragmatic as you carry forward. You've learned so much; now is the time to use that knowledge to improve your search.

KEY TAKEAWAYS

Have fun with each experience and learn as you go. Every person you meet will have traits that align with your expectations and those that don't. It's up to you where to draw the line.

Don't let an underlying health issue hold you back from having an intimate relationship. You can work around many issues by taking better care of yourself and communicating openly and honestly with your partner.

Take what you've learned so far and use it to tweak your approach as needed. Just look at what you've discovered so far and build on it.

13

CONNECTING YOUR PRESENT AND YOUR PAST

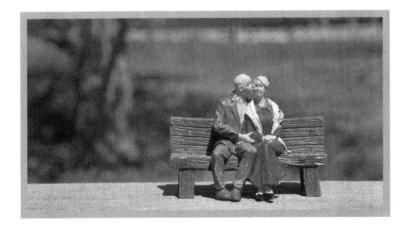

*A*s you go further along this process, life will become richer and bring more experiences and conversations that enlighten you and allow you to share your gifts with more people. It can also get a little complicated as you begin to integrate people into your social and family circles, whether it's for a short time or a more extended period. This is not stated in any way to discourage you from shaking up your world. However, it's healthy to recognize that while you may be ready for this change, the people around you may feel protective or insecure about these new developments. It's best to acknowledge them and keep them in context within the big picture of your quality of life.

Remember when you set out on this journey – or even started thinking about it, if you're still at that stage? You craved companionship and were willing to invest time and mental energy in renewing yourself and your outlook. You didn't address your past baggage – literal and figurative – just to quit because an opinionated friend, neighbor, or family member thinks a relationship is not right for you. They may be reflecting their own fears without giving it as much thought as you have.

Of course, you should listen to their concerns (if they are reasonable) and let them know that you've already schooled yourself on scams and processed your feelings regarding a past relationship. If you've had an abusive past, it's not surprising that someone who loves you wants to make sure you don't go down that unfortunate path again.

With all this in mind, this is your life. You are the one sitting home alone or holding back on booking trips because no one else will travel with you. These other people have lives of their own to make their own decisions. Don't give in to their fears and pressures.

If you need inspiration, think back on the thrill you felt when you hit a new milestone. It could have been as simple as looking at a tidier closet or admiring yourself in a mirror and really feeling proud of the changes you've made. You may have felt a rush when you posted your dating profile or received your first message, regardless of how it turned out. Those radiant moments are the ones that you have been waiting for. Relish them. Don't let anyone take them away from you.

By now, you may have found a few connections that got your heart and hopes soaring. If not, don't fret. Keep working on keeping your confidence up, since that is the greatest magnet of all. People with positive posture, a sunny smile, and sparkling conversation skills will always draw more interest. This is not about making other people happy, even those you seek out to date. This is about *you* enjoying this phase of your life unapologetically.

Just keep doing things that make you happy and good things will come. That doesn't mean retreating to your sweatpants and too many movie nights alone. The occasional break is healthy, but resist the urge to go back to your old, comfortable habits.

At this point, you may be meeting people who ask you to give in to their needs. Keep your evolving list of wants, needs, and deal-breakers nearby; don't amend them just to suit a person who only piques your interest slightly. Never settle for someone who doesn't make you truly happy. You've come too far to let someone else take the reins of your life.

Consider these individuals and how their stories worked out:

Keith was forlorn after the death of his wife, Doreen. They had been blissfully happy right up until her cancer diagnosis. Shortly after her death, his sons convinced him that he couldn't live alone as his eyesight was failing. He met up with Wenda and they got along well. She was also lonely and wanted the security of traditional marriage. They wed within a year, but found they didn't meet each other's expectations. They had never stopped to consider what they wanted, pushed by their children and the economic realities of sharing a home and an income. Their sex life was unsatisfactory, since they were not emotionally compatible. They soon found themselves living apart.

Shirley lost her husband to an affair and was devastated. She felt utterly bereft as she asked herself what she had done wrong. Bernard, who had a crush on her for years, quickly swooped in and wooed her. They also married quickly. Shirley enjoyed the chance to plan her wedding this time, since she had eloped with her first husband shortly after they discovered she was pregnant. After the glow of the wedding plans wore off, Shirley and Bernard found themselves living in an awkward dynamic where he was in love with his image of her, and she was unsure how she felt. Again, the union didn't last because they both had come into the marriage without deeply looking beyond the initial excitement.

These examples are not intended to put you off your plans. They are merely intended to show you what can happen if you settle or follow the beat of someone else's drum. At your age, you don't need someone else setting your agenda. If a person tries to push you in the wrong direction, you can stand up for your vision for your future life. That way, you won't have to start over and possibly carry more emotional scars with you.

To keep you motivated, I'll also share some happy endings:

Roberta and John always had a great professional relationship. She had left an unhappy marriage and was quite gun-shy about finding love again. John was focused on raising his sons, who were having a hard time moving out of the family nest. Ultimately, their careers took them to different towns, but they reconnected at a staff reunion. Immediately, they felt that old rapport and something more. By now, both had been journaling about what they saw in their futures and they realized the other person fit the bill. They dated long-distance for a while before Roberta moved to be closer to John and his boys. Together, they dealt with the sons' issues, drawing on Roberta's experience with her own kids. They are the best of friends and always seem to smile when they are together.

Nicole met Trevor online twelve years ago. They live in different countries but both love to travel to similar destinations. While neither one is ready to relocate, they meet twice a year on a shared vacation and have a blast. They find that they both like living independently and in locations close to their extended families. Both of them look forward to their phone and video calls but never pressure each other to switch up an arrangement that works for them.

Even if you've been single for a while and really want someone at your side, it's worthwhile to wait until the right person or people come along. A little more time alone won't break you. After all, your life is busier and more rewarding, so enjoy those fulfilling experiences for what they bring to your soul. Always focus on what you want, not on what you don't want. Stay positive and look ahead while reveling in the present. That is what life is about so be grateful for it.

ISSUES TO ADDRESS

As you settle into a relationship, or even before, you will need to think about factors beyond just your chemistry and shared interests. Depending on how the partnership evolves, you may need to discuss how you share finances or how the other person will fit in with your family and friends. This may begin with the question of who pays for the first date but goes much deeper. It reflects how you will make decisions together and what deal-breakers will influence those agreements.

Just like considering your values, these things should be considered ahead of time. Knowing what you're willing to cede and what you'll fight for will shape those discussions, hopefully in a healthy way. While where you live, and whether you will formalize your relationship are also key, finances and how your partner fits in with your family and friends are the two biggest and most complex issues people in new relationships face. Just ask any marriage counselor!

Money

This topic is a potential minefield, since it affects so many of your day-to-day decisions. At this point, you may be trying to decide whether or not to stay in your current home, if you should switch your investments to a safer strategy, or when to start claiming additional income support. These are all major factors that will play out with your long-term plans for how you will support yourself as you age.

In some couples, financial decisions are shared, while other duos delegate the tasks of bills and mortgage rates to one person. If you've been single for a while, you may wish to keep control over your money. You may not trust another person to manage your money if you've been burned before. Or you may need a hand to make a plan, if you've never lived within a budget.

People can be divided into five financial camps: high-end big spenders, money-conscious savers, unstoppable shoppers, debt-builders, and investors.[16] If you end up with a partner who is not on the same page, it could lead to heated discussions or even financial distress. It can be trickier if you have debts or feel the need to incur new ones at this point in your life.

Any respectful relationship will be based on open communication, especially on this topic. It's best to begin with recognizing the dynamics at play. Perhaps one person has the money to pay for the full cruise vacation, but their partner feels awkward not chipping in, especially if they have the funds to pay their own way. Or your new pal may be giving you investment advice that doesn't coincide with your preferred level of risk. Keep going back to your values for a reality check.

Are you turning down the cruise because you feel guilty or controlled? If the invitation was made genuinely, then ask yourself if you can move past that. Getting to the core issues behind the dollar signs will give you the insight you need to understand what is really going on.

If you end up living together, married or not, you will have a series of decisions to make about shared bills or whose name goes on a lease or a mortgage. If one person is working and the other isn't – or if one person came into the partnership with more savings – you'll want to draw up the rules before the boxes get unpacked.

This will save you from impromptu or repetitive arguments that essentially boil down to who controls what. Some couples split expenses down the middle or use ratios based on their relative earning power. Others each pick up specific items to pay for, such as groceries or utilities, after assessing the costs for their medications or alimony.

Each situation is unique. This is about emotions as much as it is about the actual dollars. If you're both financially stable and savvy, you have an easier road ahead. If you're a saver matched up with a spendaholic, then you will want to protect your finances from the other person's whims. My advice: assess where you stand and make this part of your deal-breaker list. If you cannot sort it out, meet with a neutral third party or set up your partnership in a way that allows you to be together while certain aspects of your lives are separate.

Part of the equation may be the money you share with your family or their expectations to inherit your wealth after your demise. With that in mind, here are some additional complications that can arise when you bring a new partner to meet your family.

How to Introduce Your New Mate to Your Family

If you have children, they may have a firm image of who you are and what role you should play. This is especially true if they saw you in a stable, healthy relationship with their other parent or a beloved long-time partner afterward. If they saw you escape a toxic relationship, they may hesitate to see you start over for fear that you will repeat that pattern.

You need to be aware of the origins of any doubts they express about future relationships. Then you can recognize that this is their baggage, not yours. That puts the onus back on them to resolve it, although your self-awareness can help guide them through this process.

Focus on how good this is for you. (This applies to every step that follows, by the way.)

By now, you should have given them a head's up that you're thinking about dating again. You've planted the seeds by asking them to empathize with your loneliness or boredom. That should help them to understand *why* you are interested in pursuing a new partnership. You can share those details about what type of relationship you're pursuing, if you think it will ease their worries. You're not obligated to tell them anything; your family dynamics will dictate how much you will impart, knowing that information tends to migrate through a family grapevine quickly. By telling people directly, you control the message.

Once you meet someone you plan to spend quite a bit of time with, you'll have to decide when to loop your new partner into the family. It's easier to start with allies rather than doubters. Smaller introductions are less stressful for everyone, compared to bringing them to a wedding where they get bombarded with names and faces. You can either begin with your closest relatives or those who will be most accepting. Whatever you need to feel safe and supported is the most vital at this crucial juncture.

Keep initial meetings low-key and have an activity planned so you don't end up standing around waiting for someone to fill the conversational void. Even if you're passionate in person, don't touch each other beyond hand-holding yet. Instead, emphasize everyone's common ground and encourage them to get to know each other better. Make sure you still make time for your family members to see you on your own as well, especially in the early days. They may be naturally jealous to 'lose you' to someone else, so give them time.

Just like money issues, the tension may come down to a sense of control. Reassure your loved ones that you are still in charge of your life, but this person is part of your present. If you start making changes, such as moving or traveling more, your family may worry that your decisions are being influenced by your partner. To keep the peace, present a united front and be clear that you are doing what you want with the love and support of your partner. If you attribute too many reasons to "Drew thinks we should do this," you'll fuel concerns that this new person is steering you away from your usual approach and over-ruling your regular network.

Take it slow. Give them time to adjust. Explain what is happening and why from your perspective. Accept that this change is new to them, and they may not be as ready as you are to embrace it.

If they count on you for certain things – child care or hosting holiday dinners, for example – don't disrupt those traditions lightly. Reassure people with your actions that you are still part of their team too. If they have concerns, talk them through. However, don't allow them to place your needs beyond theirs. That is as unhealthy as letting your partner do it.

Remind the people who love you that you're safe and following a path that you have mapped out for your happiness. That should give them enough reason to come aboard.

Wow! Can you believe that you've gone from thinking about dating to planning how to introduce a new partner to your family? If you have followed the steps in each chapter, you should be very close to this exciting point. Don't rush it if it's taken longer than you've expected. Good things are ahead, thanks to the work you've done to bring out the best in wonderful you.

* * *

WEEK 12 ASSIGNMENTS

❖ Keep doing the habits from Weeks 1 to 11 that sustain you and keep you on track. Explore the world via social outings, books, conversations, and online experiences.

❖ Write in your journal how proud you are of how far you have come and how much stronger and happier you may feel now. This applies whether you're with a potential mate or still single.

❖ Take an "after" picture of yourself, both a headshot and a full-body shot, then compare it to when you first started this twelve-week plan. It's not so much about how much skinnier you feel; it's the brightness in your eyes and smile that counts.

❖ Congratulate yourself on how far you've come!

KEY TAKEAWAYS

Refine your search based on what you want. Never settle for less than what you truly deserve. You've worked too hard to backslide.

Money issues will lead to conflict unless you openly discuss your financial personality, any previous money problems, and how you wish to share your resources in your new life together.

Your family will respond better to a new partner if you address their concerns and show them how this new relationship is good for you. Allay their fears and reassure them that you're not leaving every aspect of your previous life behind.

CONCLUSION

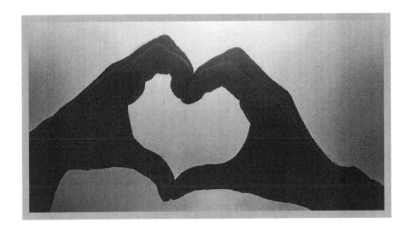

*A*s scary as it can feel to push ourselves out of our comfort zones, the payoff is worth that initial unease. With regular doses of belief in yourself and work to clean your slate (and your environment), you open yourself up to new possibilities for the years ahead. Not only will you have renewed confidence and a stronger sense of your priorities, but chances are also very good that you will – or have already – attracted a partner who contributes to them too.

Enjoy every moment.

If your situation changes, you are still equipped to pick yourself back up and realize that you can move on. That resilience will serve you well in many areas of your life. Embrace it.

By now, you should be healthier from getting out and moving your body. You have created a more robust social network by joining activities and meeting new people. At a time when many people are losing their friends, you are reversing that trend. That is golden on its own.

You have also challenged yourself to learn new skills and generate a refreshed outlook, not only about yourself but who you want in your life. What felt so daunting a few weeks ago should be second nature by now after all the practice you have done to initiate conversations and to venture to new places.

As we age, we tend to fall into familiar patterns, which require less brainpower to get through the days. Again, you are defying the perceived constraints of your age and living your days richly. You should now have a slightly higher appetite for small risks that may have intimidated you before. Use that confidence to keep growing as a person.

Having lived this journey myself, I want you to remember what you have learned and to continue to use it to create a happy and fulfilling life in whatever way works for you; I know that you can do this.

Now, get out there and enjoy what you have learned. The world is rich with amazing people, places, and experiences. There is no reason why you shouldn't enjoy it and enrich it for others. Go spread some smiles and joy.

The more positive you are, the more you will smile. That triggers your 'happy hormones' to dance with more enthusiasm in your brain, lowering your stress levels, and making you even more buoyant. Now, that is a chemistry that you can really enjoy... until you connect with someone who offers a different type of chemistry.

Stay safe, optimistic, and informed. Yes, there are bad people out there. There are also countless good people who want the same things you do. It may take a little effort to find them and build a relationship. By consistently doing the things we've covered, more of them will come to light.

Be realistic and you will be fine. You are now more aware of how scammers and other manipulators operate, so your guard will be up as you watch for warning signs. Share that knowledge with others as you continue to be a positive force in the world.

If you wish to keep the conversation rolling, you are personally invited by me to join our private community Facebook group, entitled Vibrant Living – Aging Well. I post articles, tips, and tools on all aspects of vibrant living and aging well and love hearing back from clients and readers. You can also meet some dynamic people like yourself who are on a similar journey.

If you enjoyed this book, please don't be shy about saying so. My goal is to help as many people as possible to find happiness within themselves and with others. So please share this title with your friends and leave a review wherever you purchased this book, so more amazing humans can find love, companionship, or a travel buddy of their own.

We all crave personal relationships that make us feel special. Now that you are one step closer, let's keep the momentum going!

TWELVE-WEEK PROGRAM

_T_his section provides you space to track your progress and capture your steps in one easy spot. If you need more sheets – and I hope you do – then simply add some loose-leaf notes to write down the thoughts and experiences that keep you motivated.

WEEK 1 ASSIGNMENTS

❖ Take a few pictures of yourself, including a headshot and an image of your full body. If you're not used to being on this end of the lens, don't be shy. Just do it so we can compare your photo now to one that you will take at the end of the twelve-week program. Check off a box each time you add one to the collection.

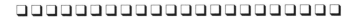

❖ Sit down and brainstorm all the words that describe who you are. The core values exercise may help you get started, but let's build on it. Seek out neutral or positive words, such as friendly, heart-centred, chatty, trustworthy, etc. Write them in your journal. This will not be a definitive list. You will build on it as we go through each week.

For example: Friendly	

WEEK 2 ASSIGNMENTS

❖ By now, you've got a great start on your list of positive attributes about yourself, so keep going! Now that you know what you want, you can think about words that fit that model. For example, you may feel you are loyal or free-spirited. As long as you are honest, that's what matters.

❖ Next, you will write a short letter about a past relationship. This letter is for your eyes only. If your ex is still around, do not mail it or share anything about it on social media. Simply say 'thank you' for the past experience and all the learning, but acknowledge that you are now moving on. If your partner has passed away, write a short letter (if you can) about how much you miss them and reassure them that you are continuing your life in a positive way, while making the decision to attract new people into your life. If you can't write the words, then say them out loud in a heartfelt way. Whichever situation you are in, tell that person how you have great optimism that your life will only be better from this point forward.

👋 Give yourself a mental high-five when you're done!

WEEK 3 ASSIGNMENTS

❖ Choose one room or closet to declutter this week. Specify which day and time you will tackle it so you don't procrastinate. Once you get going, I'll bet you find it invigorating, so keep going. It's truly amazing what we keep around when we don't have our radar attuned to this task. Check off a box each time you clear one more space.

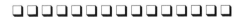

❖ Find some form of movement, such as walking, hitting the treadmill, doing yoga, stretching, or strength training, that you will perform twenty to thirty minutes

147

a day. Start slow and enjoy the feeling of your body getting stronger and more limber each day. If you need to, schedule it as well.

Form of Exercise	Duration

Pat yourself on the back when you finish your first session. (Hey, that's also a stretch so you can count it as exercise!)

❖ Continue adding positive words to describe yourself in your journal. Keep looking for ways to celebrate your good traits so you are reminded of just how precious you are. It's okay if you accidentally repeat some words. That just makes you doubly awesome!

WEEK 4 ASSIGNMENTS

❖ Carry on with the tasks from Weeks 1 to 3. Keep documenting your attributes, sorting through the detritus of your life, and exercising your body.

❖ Add in the kind deeds you do for others and the books you have been reading. Looking back on this list (and the one above) should make you feel like you are shedding your own skin so a new one shines through.

Books	Kind deeds

❖ Choose one or two inspirational quotes and one or two inspirational affirmations that you will write out and place on your bathroom wall, in your office, or on the fridge as a daily reminder of what is important in your life.

Quotes/Affirmations

WEEK 5 ASSIGNMENTS

❖ Carry on with the tasks from Weeks 1 to 4. Keep writing down your good points, trying new exercises, and tackling one more closet or drawer to toss out clutter.

❖ As more inspirational quotes and affirmations come into view (this is where your Reticular Activating System comes in handy), add them to your home to keep your spirits up and your mind planning for brighter days ahead.

❖ Draft your list of wants, needs, and deal-breakers without capping it off. More ideas will pop up as we work through the next steps. Keep an open mind at all times.

Wants	Needs	Deal-breakers

WEEK 6 ASSIGNMENTS

❖ Carry on with the tasks from Weeks 1 to 5. Keep flattering yourself by writing good points in your journal, exercising regularly, and clearing out old baggage.

❖ Add more inspirational quotes and affirmations as they come to you, and enjoy each one.

❖ Keep your list of wants, needs, and deal-breakers handy as you watch other couples – real or fictional – to determine what resonates with you.

❖ Every day, find a chance to chat with someone in your circle. If you don't see people in person, dial up an old friend to see how they are.

❖ Check off a box for every friend you reach out to:

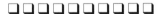

❖ Set up one to two events this week, such as meeting a friend (new or old) or relative for coffee, a walk, or a casual meal. As one event ends, plan where you want to go next to keep up the momentum. Start stockpiling ideas, since you will be continuing this trend from now until the end of the program. Circle one of the symbols below every time you get out of the house with a friend. By the time you've circled them all, this habit will be firmly in place.

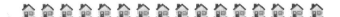

WEEK 7 ASSIGNMENTS

❖ Carry on with the tasks from Weeks 1 to 6. Keep writing in your journal, getting out to exercise, and seeking out positive affirmations.

❖ Keep reading, being grateful, and seeking ways to get out of the house to spread joy to people around you.

Attributes	Books	Gratitude

❖ Commit to joining one regular activity outside of the house. You've already gone out for lunch, but now you need a club or a course to learn something new and connect with people in a shared setting. There are endless possibilities, so keep an open mind. Circle one club below as you try out a new, regular activity. Stick with it until you find one(s) that fits.

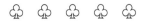

WEEK 8 ASSIGNMENTS

❖ Carry on with the tasks from Weeks 1 to 7. Stay positive and active as you embrace new places and opportunities.

❖ Find new books to read and new faces to pepper with compliments. Your mind and your circle of influence should be growing.

❖ Keep finding reasons to leave the house and meet new people. Identify target-rich environments and go there regularly to interact with people. Don't be too shy or you'll defeat your purpose of going out in the first place.

❖ Get a current photo of yourself while out doing activities you enjoy. You can hire a professional photographer, take a selfie, or ask a friend or relative to help you. Choose a setting that makes you smile, preferably in natural light that flatters you.

☺ Smile! You have lots of reasons to beam your positivity far and wide.

WEEK 9 ASSIGNMENTS

❖ Carry on with the tasks from Weeks 1 to 8. Keep focusing on staying active, in terms of exercising and socializing with friends and weekly activities.

❖ Read new books and watch out for more inspirational posts to keep you energized. By now, these habits should be part of your routine as you continue to learn about yourself and the world around you.

❖ Keep seeking out target-rich places to shop and spend your social time. Try new stores, even if you're just browsing. Ask your friends where they see people like the mates you are seeking and follow their advice. By now, people should know you're up for dating, so make them your allies (and your scouts.)

❖ Create your online dating profile without overthinking it. Have fun with your drafts and pick out the photos that you feel portray the inner you. You can tweak it after the first draft but take that first step to figure out which platforms work for you and how they work. Again, you will learn as you go.

Platform	Research for suitability	Profile created
eHarmony		
Match		
Silver Singles		
Senior Match		
Our Time		
Other		

WEEK 10 ASSIGNMENTS

❖ Carry on with the tasks from Weeks 1 to 9. On top of the fun things listed in the previous paragraph, tackle new book titles and keep your energy up with exercise and aspirations.

❖ Keep visiting target-rich places in case you meet an intriguing person there. If you don't, you're still honing your conversation skills that you can use in other settings.

❖ Update your online dating profile based on any points that seem to resonate with people when they message you. Add more fun photos as you add to your collection. This will give your fans new material to admire.

Platform	Profile updated	New photos added
eHarmony		
Match		
Silver Singles		
Senior Match		
Our Time		
Other		

❖ Keep track of how much time you spend on your online dating activities. It's surprising how time can slip away. If it's more than an hour a day, dial it back. Taking a balanced approach is better for you in the long run.

Day	Time spent	Day	Time spent
1		7	
2		8	
3		9	
4		10	
5		11	
6		12	

WEEK 11 ASSIGNMENTS

❖ Carry on with the tasks from Weeks 1 to 10. By now you should be naturally finding and clearing items you don't need while picking up books and inspirational quotes effortlessly. Keep focusing on removing parts of your unwanted past as you build your brain for an optimistic future.

❖ Get out of the house to enjoy people and activities that infuse you with life, especially areas and interests that may have you crossing paths with a sexy new partner.

❖ Check in on your online dating network daily unless you feel like you need to pause to develop something deeper with one person – either in person or online. Only you will know when to stop shopping, but it doesn't hurt to look around, as long as you're only having dates on a superficial level. Once things get more intense, you'll have to make a decision.

Platform	Number of messages	Keep or Abandon?
eHarmony		
Match		
Silver Singles		
Senior Match		
Our Time		
Other		

❖ Reassess your wants, needs, and deal-breaker lists as you meet people and discover how much they still fit their respective categories. Maybe your online matches have opened your eyes to how much you had committed to sticking to your guns. Based on your experience, you may wish to tighten the rules or bend them a little more. This is a good time to do a reality check so you can be more pragmatic as you carry forward. You've learned so much; now is the time to use that knowledge to improve your search.

Wants	Needs	Deal-breakers

WEEK 12 ASSIGNMENTS

❖ Review and keep doing the habits from Weeks I to II that sustain you and keep you on track. Explore the world via social outings, books, conversations, and online experiences.

❖ Write in your journal how proud you are of how far you have come, and how much stronger and happier you may feel now. This applies whether you're with a potential mate or still single.

❖ Take an "after" picture of yourself, both a headshot and a full-body shot, then compare it to when you first started this twelve-week plan. It's not so much about how much skinnier you feel; it's the brightness in your eyes and smile that counts.

❖ Congratulate yourself on how far you've come!

FROM THE AUTHOR

Thank you so much for reading *The Art of Senior Dating*. Please don't forget to write a brief review wherever you purchased this book. I am grateful for all feedback and your review will help other readers decide whether to read this book too. Follow this link to leave a review:

Interested in staying in touch to hear about any of my future books or projects? Would you like the opportunity to work with me directly in a personalized 90-day program?

Contact me at ravina@ravinachandra.com

or visit www.ravinachandra.com

PSSSST, DON'T FORGET YOUR FREE GIFT!

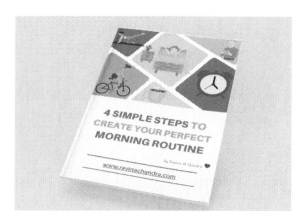

In '**4 Simple Steps to Create Your Perfect Morning Routine,**' you will discover:

- What a **morning routine** is and why it is essential you have one
- Why having a morning routine will bring you **more focus, productivity, and purpose to your life**
- The secret of creating a morning routine using these **four components** that will **align with your core values**
- How a morning routine can elevate your life so that you may live **vibrantly,** whether you are seeking a companion, exploring new interests, or improving your health

Go to www.ravinachandra.com/books to get it NOW

ENDNOTES

Chapter 1 Resources
The Top 10 Things Men In Their 50s Want In A Woman, https://www.singleandmature.com/the-top-10-things-men-in-their-50s-want-in-a-woman

Brown, Susan and Wright, Matthew, Marriage, Cohabitation, and Divorce in Later Life, *Innovation in Aging*, Volume 1, Issue 2, September 2017, https://academic.oup.com/innovateage/article/1/2/igx015/4157719

Chapter 7 Resources:
GetSetUp: Live Online Classes for Older Adults, https://www.getsetup.io

Chapter 10 Resources
Manning, Margaret, The Top 5 Best Dating Sites for Seniors, blog post, Aug. 6, 2020, Sixtyandme.com, https://sixtyandme.com/best-senior-dating-sites/

Chapter 11 Resources

Khan, Khalid, and Chaudry, Sameer, An evidence-based approach to an ancient pursuit: a systematic review on converting online contact into a first date, BMJ Evidence-Based Medicine, Feb. 12, 2015, https://ebm.bmj.com/content/20/2/48

Chapter 13 Resources

McWhinney, Jamie, Top 6 Marriage-Killing Money Issues: How to Keep Them from Damaging Your Relationship, Investopedia blog, June 15, 2021, https://www.investopedia.com/articles/pf/09/marriage-killing-money-issues.asp

Introducing Your Children to a New Partner, Better Relationships blog post, Jan. 7, 2021, https://www.betterrelationships.org.au/family-parenting/blended-families/introducing-your-new-partner/

REFERENCES

1. Cherlin, A. J. (2010). Demographic trends in the United States: A review of research in the 2000s. Journal of Marriage and Family, 72, 403–419.

2. Uhlenberg, P., and Myers, M. A. P. (1981). Divorce and the elderly. The Gerontologist, 21, 276–282.

3. Sundberg, L. et al. (2018). Why is the gender gap in life expectancy decreasing? The impact of age- and cause-specific mortality in Sweden 1997–2014, April 2018, https://www.ncbi.nlm.nih.gov/pmc/articles/PMC6015620/

4. Physical Activity and Health: A Report of the Surgeon General, Older Adults, Centers for Disease Control and Prevention, United States, https://www.cdc.gov/nccdphp/sgr/olderad.htm

5. Merle, A. The Reading Habits of Ultra-Successful

People, The Huffington Post, Dec. 6, 2017, https://www.huff post.com/entry/the-reading-habits-of-ult_b_9688130

6. Brown, J. and Wong, J. How Gratitude Changes You and Your Brain, Greater Good Magazine, June 6, 2017, https:// greatergood.berkeley.edu/article/item/ how_gratitude_changes_you_and_your_brain

7. Calasanti, T., and Kiecolt, K. J. (2007). Diversity among late life couples. *Generations: Journal of the American Society on Aging*, 31, 10–17.

8. Brown, S. L., Lin, I. F., Hammersmith, A. M., & Wright, M. R. (2016). Later life marital dissolution and repartner-ship status: A national portrait. Series B, Volume 73, issue 6, p. 1032-1042. *Journals of Gerontology: Social Sciences.* doi:10.1093/geronb/gbw051

9. Federal Trade Commission, (2019). What You Need to Know About Romance Scams, https://www.consumer.ftc. gov/articles/what-you-need-know-about-romance-scams

10. How to Land Your Man, by Dr. Phil's staff, via his blog, Dec. 6, 2005, https://www.drphil.com/advice/how-to-land-your-man/

11. Love Smart: Part 2 - Target-Rich Environments, by Dr. Phil's staff, via his blog, (2021). https://www.drphil.com/ slideshows/love-smart-part-2-target-rich-environments/

12. Lee, J. 26 Dating Profile Examples, blog post on

HealthyFramework.com, https://healthyframework.com/
dating/beginners/dating-profile-examples/

13. Stein, L. Sex and Seniors: the 70-Year-Itch, the Health
Day blog, June 12, 2021, https://consumer.healthday.com/
encyclopedia/aging-1/misc-aging-news-10/sex-and-
seniors-the-70-year-itch-647575.html

14. Karram, M. Three Things Women Need to Know
About Pelvic Floor Disorders, The Christ Church Health
Network, blog post, May 11, 2020, https://www.
thechristhospital.com/healthspirations/3-things-women-
need-to-know-about-pelvic-floor-disorders

15. Maiorino, M., et al. (2015) Lifestyle modifications and
erectile dysfunction. Asian Journal of Andrology, January-
February 2015, Volume 17, issue 1, p. 5-10. https://www.ncbi.
nlm.nih.gov/pmc/articles/PMC4291878/

16. Smith, L. What Is Your Money Personality? Investopedia blog post, updated July 21, 2021, https://www.investo
pedia.com/articles/basics/07/money-personality.asp

IMAGE CREDITS

Chapter 1: 1950s photo courtesy of efes, Pixabay.com, Pixabay License

Chapter 2: Contemplative Senior photo courtesy of CaroleGomez, Canva.com, One Design Use License Agreement

Chapter 3: Photo courtesy of Natalie Grainger, Unsplash.com, Unsplash License

Chapter 4: Photo courtesy of Becca McHaffie, Unsplash.com, Unsplash License; Move those Muscles photo courtesy of Anupam Mahapatra, Unsplash.com, Unsplash License

Chapter 5: Photo by Geralt, Pixabay.com, Pixabay.com, Pixabay License

Chapter 6: Photo courtesy of Creative-Family, Canva.com, One Design Use License

Chapter 7: Photo courtesy of Brett Jordan, Unsplash.com, Unsplash License

Chapter 8: Photo courtesy of Markus Winkler, Unspash.com, Unsplash License

Chapter 9: Group of Senior Friends photo courtesy of Monkey Business Images, Canva.com, One Design Use License

Chapter 10: Photo courtesy of athree23, Pixabay.com, Pixabay License

Chapter 11: Photo by Joshua Hoehne, Unsplash.com, Unsplash License

Chapter 12: Romantic Senior Couple photo by aldomurillo, Canva.com, One Design Use License

Chapter 13: Photo courtesy of Erika Wittlieb, Pixabay.com, Pixabay License

Conclusion: Photo courtesy of Saiph Muhammad, Unsplash.com, Unsplash License.

Printed in Great Britain
by Amazon

31451962R00106